Celebrating Life Decades After Breast Cancer

40 Women Share Stories of Surviving
Twenty to Fifty Years After Diagnosis

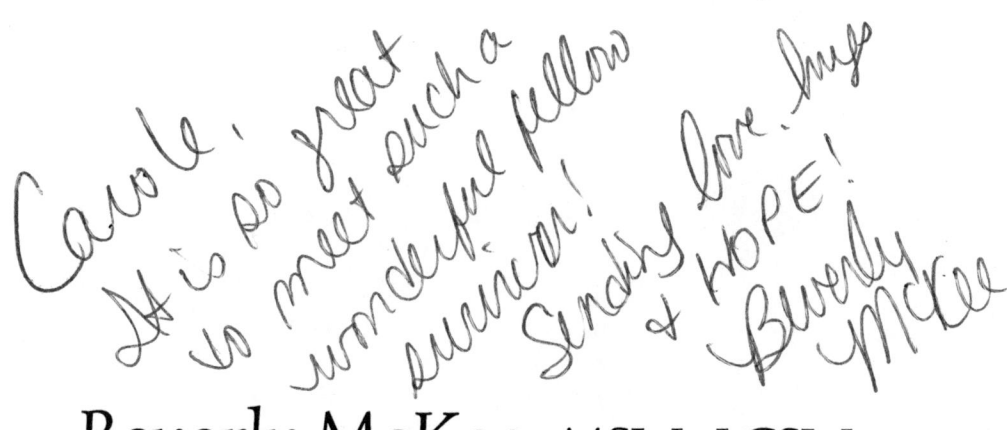

Beverly McKee, MSW, LCSW

Transformation Media Books
Bloomington, Indiana

Copyright © 2015 Beverly McKee & Navigating the Storms, LLC

All rights reserved. No part of this book may be reproduced or transmitted in any form or by any means, electronic or mechanical, including photocopying, recording, or by any information storage and retrieval system, without permission in writing from the publisher.

Published by Transformation Media Books, USA

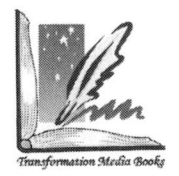

www.TransformationMediaBooks.com
info@TransformationMediaBooks.com

An imprint of Pen & Publish, Inc.
www.PenandPublish.com
Bloomington, Indiana
(314) 827-6567

Print ISBN: 978-1-941799-17-8
eBook ISBN: 978-1-941799-18-5

Cover Design: Jennifer Geist
Cover Artwork: Bolina, via 123RF Stock Photo
Author Photo: Angela Rue, Rue 2 Photography

For Dan, Jack, and Alex

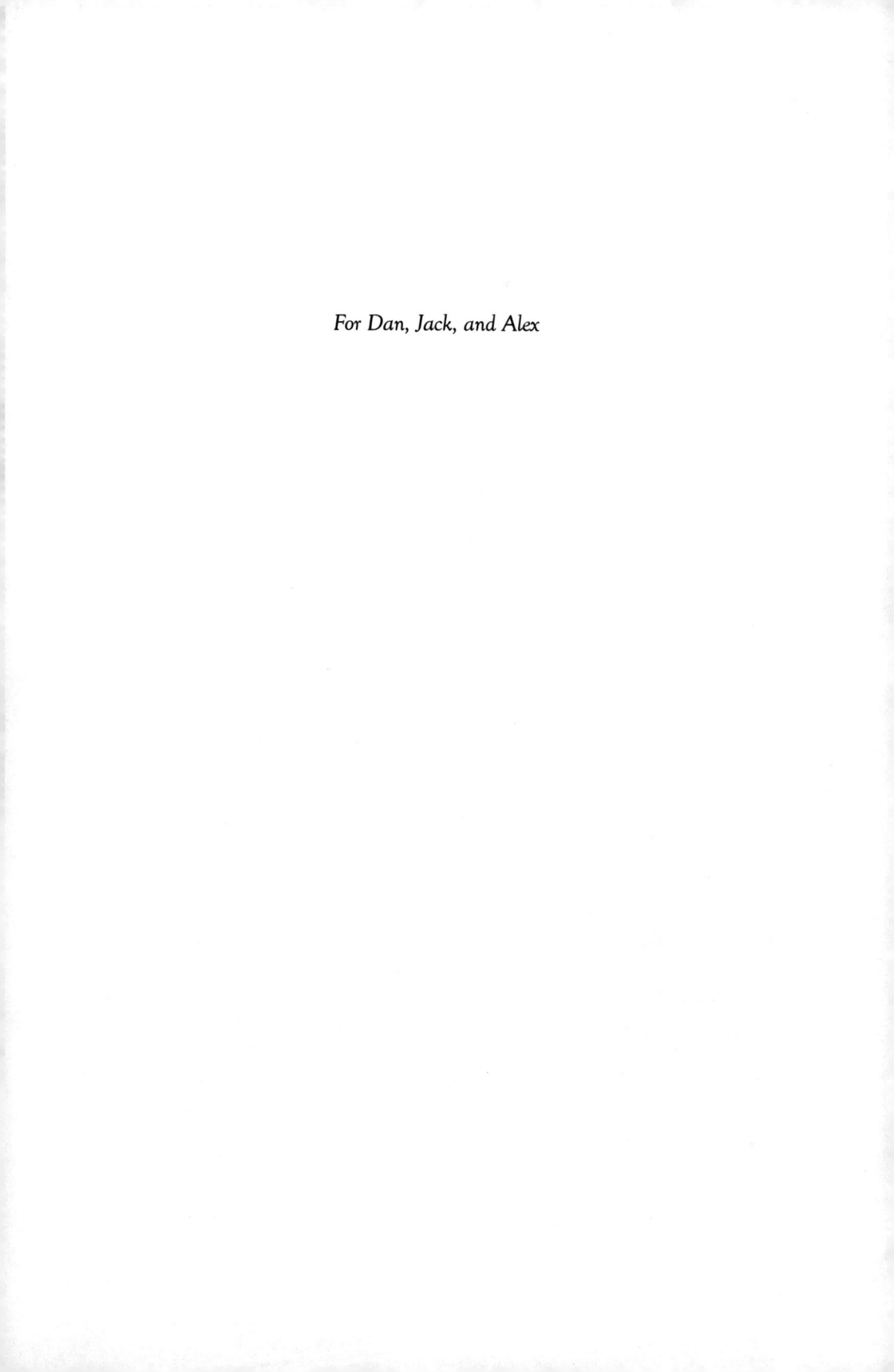

Contents

Prologue 7
Introduction 9

Section 1
Breast Cancer as a Catalyst for Change

Chapter 1 | Anne Erikson 15
Chapter 2 | Nancy Bruning 21
Chapter 3 | Barbara Cunnings-Versaevel 25
Chapter 4 | Bobbi de Cordova-Hanks 29
Chapter 5 | Ginny Mason 35
Chapter 6 | Beverly Vote 43
Chapter 7 | Karen Eubanks Jackson 47
Chapter 8 | Eunice Walker 51
Chapter 9 | Chris Mulder 57
Chapter 10 | Marilyn Fries 61
Chapter 11 | Odell Sauls 65

Section 2
The Power of a Positive Attitude

Chapter 12 | Carolyn Smith 71
Chapter 13 | Jo McCall 75
Chapter 14 | Mary Ellen Koch 79
Chapter 15 | Erin Jones 85
Chapter 16 | Margaret Blades 91
Chapter 17 | Rhonda Chavis 95
Chapter 18 | Cheryl Coomes 99
Chapter 19 | Rosalind Steel 103
Chapter 20 | Lisa Cushing 107
Chapter 21 | Tonya Salkowski 111

Section 3
Faith in God, Self, and Others

Chapter 22 | Grace Allen 117
Chapter 23 | Marsha Polys 121
Chapter 24 | Francis Putney 127
Chapter 25 | Gail Plude 131
Chapter 26 | May Newman 135
Chapter 27 | Sherry Suon 139
Chapter 28 | Carol Smith 145
Chapter 29 | Patti Nacci 149
Chapter 30 | Jayne Bailey 153

Section 4
Defying the Odds

Chapter 31 | Dr. Jacqueline Kerr 159
Chapter 32 | Marianne Werton 165
Chapter 33 | Linda Radick 171
Chapter 34 | Debbie Davis 175
Chapter 35 | Beverly Hunter Anderson 179
Chapter 36 | Corky Ellis 185
Chapter 37 | Ellen Frketic 189
Chapter 38 | Mary Rath 193
Chapter 39 | Stephanie Smith 197
Chapter 40 | You'll Have to Read It to Believe It! 203

Sneak Peek 207
Acknowledgments 209
About Beverly McKee 211

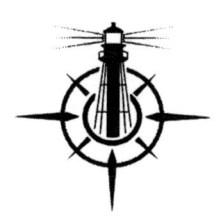

PROLOGUE

Survival instinct pulls her from sleep. Danger is lurking in the room . . . constricting her lungs. Her body screams for oxygen but she is too afraid to breathe. Every muscle stands on alert, ready to bolt from the danger at hand, her brain processing the silence. Cold sweat rolls down her cheeks, eyes wide with fear. What woke her?

Stark, cold reality sinks into her pores as the source of her fear rears its ugly head. Salty tears mix with perspiration, covering her cheeks. The danger is imminent but there is no escape, nowhere to hide. The four words that set off this chain reaction echoing throughout her brain: "You have breast cancer." Leaving the comfort of her bed, she longs for the safety of her new friends . . . forty women who surround her with HOPE and insight into surviving breast cancer for twenty, thirty, forty, even fifty years. She curls up with a blanket and her copy of Celebrating Life Decades after Breast Cancer, *absorbing the stories that quiet the fear, calm the anxiety, and offer the priceless gift of HOPE.*

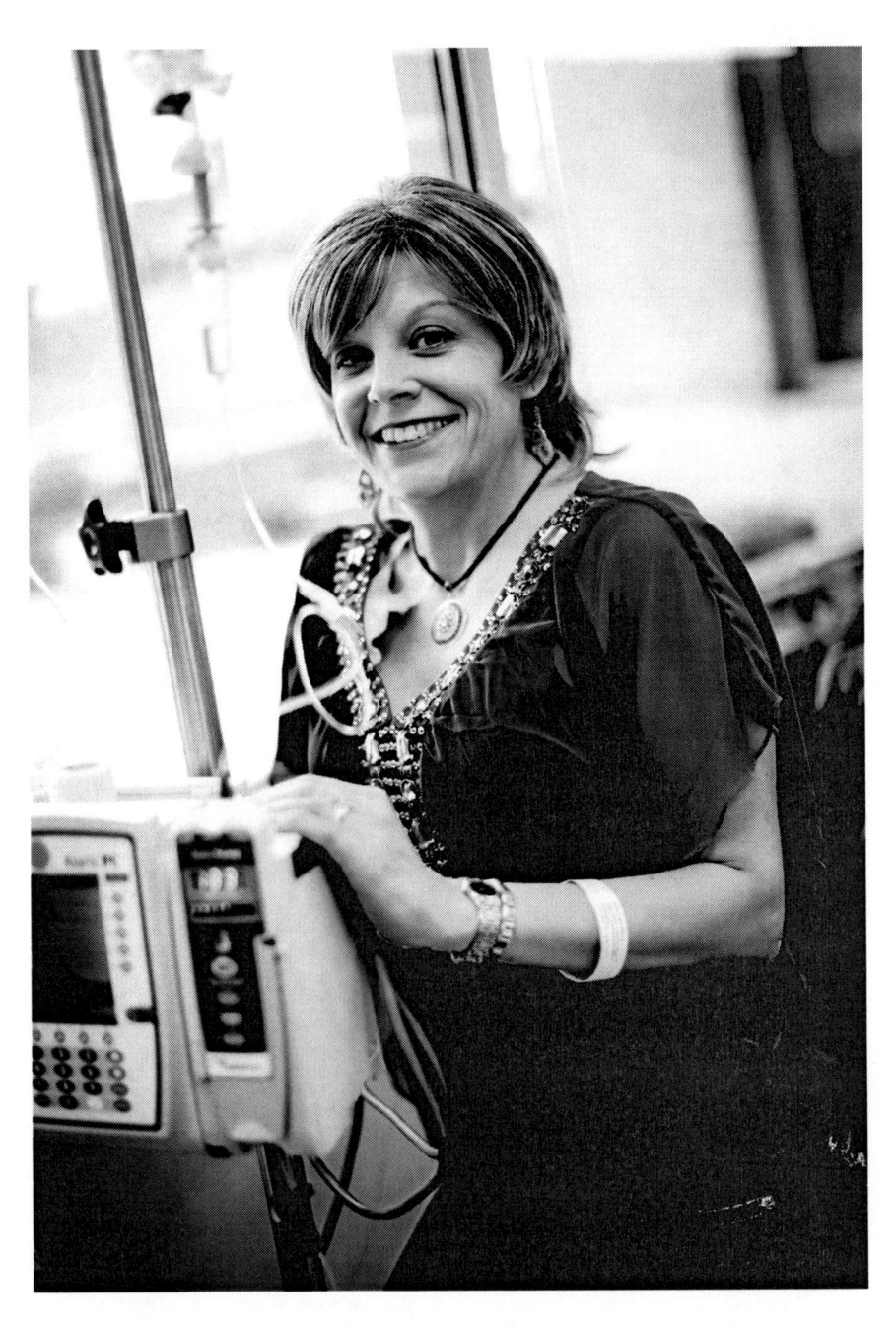

Beverly during one of eight chemotherapy treatments in 2012

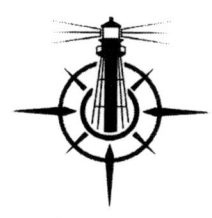

INTRODUCTION

Breast cancer survivors and their loved ones throughout the world can relate to the internal struggle that comes from living with this disease . . . it is a unique, inescapable dilemma. I know, because I was the woman in that story not so long ago. I heard those words on October 17, 2012, at 4:25 pm.

"You have breast cancer."

Every ounce of my security was shattered . . . tiny shards of glass falling all around me. I was vulnerable and felt very alone as mortality knocked on my door. Moments after that call, my boys walked in from school with three friends. Their innocent laughter forcing me into autopilot: make dinner, empty the dishwasher, fold the laundry. Welcomed distractions from the new concept dancing in my brain . . . breast cancer was growing inside of me. It was too much to absorb all at once.

Nightfall brought darkness and solitude. With sweet dreams well beyond reach, I left my fitfully sleeping husband to check on my innocent boys. My heart ached at the thought of sharing my news with them. By noon the next day, I found myself in the waiting room of my oncologist's office. Our conversation would be a catalyst for this book, sparked by an idea born in a stark white oncology office.

A new world of terminology flooded my brain. Invasive lobular carcinoma, bilateral mastectomy, chemotherapy, radiation, recurrence, metastasis. Four words, "You have breast cancer" had set me on this course but now four new words would shape my future: "five-year-survival rates." Those words echoing throughout the recesses of my brain. "Five-year-survival rates!" I pictured my little boys . . . they wouldn't be old enough to drive in five years. I felt compelled to interrupt my oncologist.

"With all due respect, Dr. O., I don't care about five-year-survival rates.

What do I need to do to survive breast cancer for forty years?"

She stopped, mid-sentence, laughed out loud, and we agreed to take an aggressive approach to treatment. A licensed mental health therapist by training and an optimist at heart, I went home and planned a party. A celebration forty years into the future on the anniversary of my diagnosis . . . please consider this your official invitation to my "40-Year Survivor Celebration":

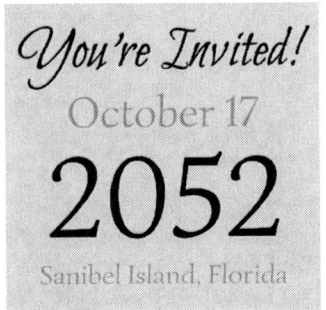

You're Invited!
October 17
2052
Sanibel Island, Florida

Sleepless nights gave me ample time to plan the party details. Candles on white tablecloths, blowing in the salty ocean breeze, surrounded by my family and friends. A new determination replaced anxiety, but I needed true-life examples that would guide me on my journey.

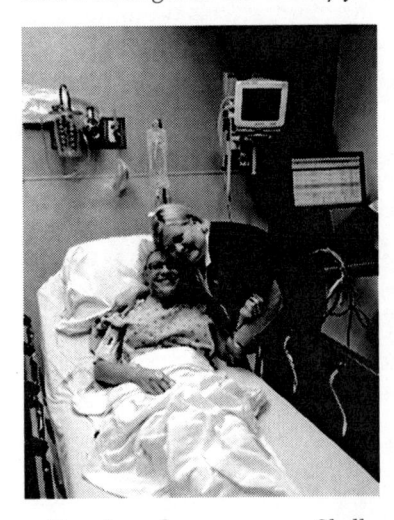

Beverly and surgery nurse Shelly

Preparing for a bilateral mastectomy with reconstruction, I engaged in a desperate quest to find a book about long-term breast cancer survivors. I wanted inspiration and insight from women who had accomplished my new life mission: to survive breast cancer for decades. My fingers tapping the keyboard frantically as every search ended with the same unfathomable result. There were no books like this one. It didn't make sense to me. I knew the survivors were out there and I needed to hear their stories to get through the dark days. And so began my journey to write this book . . . for myself, for the five million breast cancer survivors throughout the world, their loved ones and the oncology teams that help us heal on a daily basis.

As the effects of chemotherapy, multiple surgeries and radiation took their toll on my body, the book took on a life of its own. A worldwide search through my website/blog www.navigating.org, social media, word of mouth, oncology offices, public speaking events and TV/radio appearances brought us together . . . phenomenal women with stories to share about thriving decades after diagnosis. Forty interviews, one for every year that I plan to survive until my big celebration on the beach.

These inspiring women opened their hearts and souls, opening old wounds by discussing their day of diagnosis from twenty, thirty, forty, and for some, even fifty years ago. Emotional conversations lasted for hours, discussing that fateful day that unite us in a strong sisterhood. Every story is as unique as the women themselves. They come from all over the world with different types of breast cancer, at every stage including Stage IV, at different points in life.

The struggle with breast cancer is universal but coping mechanisms are unique for everyone, based on life experience, external support systems, and our outlook on the future. You'll recognize yourself in many of the stories and struggles as each woman shares her intimate journey through diagnosis and treatment. Many were encouraged to get their affairs in order as their prognosis was undeniably grim. Each holiday and family event met with a plethora of mixed emotions: sheer joy for being alive to witness it in contrast to stark fear that it would be their last. They moved past treatment one day, one month, one year at a time, thrilled to watch their children moving into adulthood and spoiling grandchildren they never believed they would meet. Weakened at times with the fear and anxiety that cuts deep into the soul, they leaned heavily on their faith and loved ones. For many, a new passion was born out of the storm of breast cancer. Their lives and careers set in the course of a new direction.

Each woman shares her insight and reflections into why she has survived for decades after diagnosis, but there is no magic cure hidden among these pages. They share the commonality of facing their own mortality too soon in life. A hard lesson, perhaps, but truth be told, all of us must accept this universal truth at some point.

No one is disputing that breast cancer has a dark side, but each of these stories helped me heal the hidden wounds of breast cancer. I'm a changed person because of these women and now you are invited to become immersed in this community of like-minded survivors in a land of HOPE and inspiration. It is a great privilege to share their stories with you and the entire world.

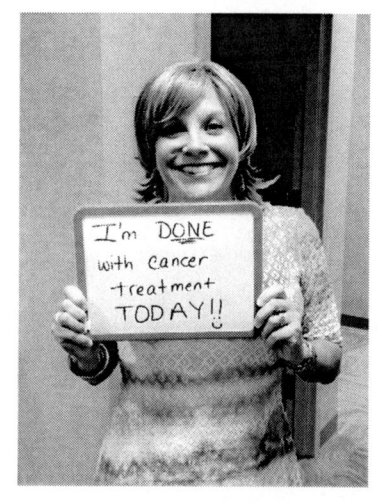

A day of celebration!

I welcome you to join me on my website, www.navigating.org, to learn how you can meet the inspirational women from this book on my worldwide book tour, join an exclusive online book club and to stay up to date about future book releases.

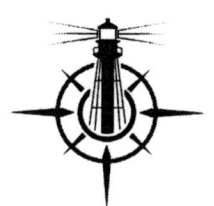

Section 1

Breast Cancer as a Catalyst for Change

The four words, "You have breast cancer," initiate women into a life-changing club that no one wants to join. Many of the women in this book have used their diagnoses as a catalyst for positive change in their lives, thereby improving the lives of breast cancer survivors throughout the world.

Stories include changing career paths to become advocates for breast cancer survivors, starting support groups, exercise programs, mastectomy shops, magazines, and resource centers. On a more personal level, some of the women left unhealthy relationships or unsatisfying careers after their diagnoses, enjoying long, happy, healthy lives decades later.

Their stories may inspire you to make a change in your life!

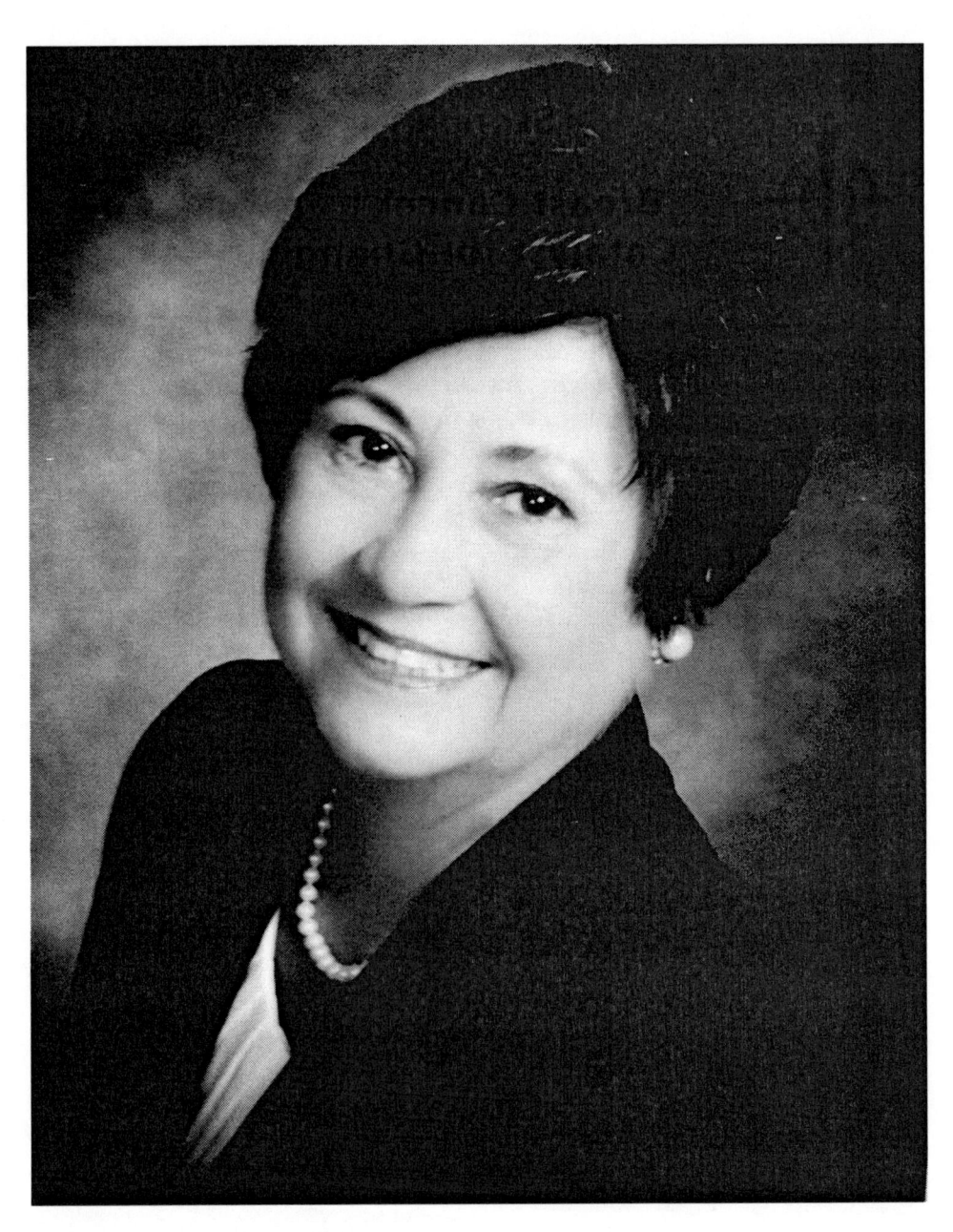

Anne celebrating life decades after breast cancer!

CHAPTER 1 | Anne Erikson

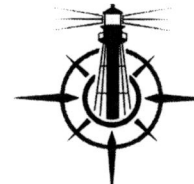

Celebrating Life Since She Was Diagnosed
in October 1974
White Creek, TN

"I never felt like less of a woman because of my mastectomy. What bothered me was the isolation. Breast cancer was so secretive forty-one years ago and support was not visible."

Anne was in the midst of the sandwich generation, searching for that delicate balance between being a single mom to two boys, ages twelve and seven, and helping care for her father who was battling cancer. She didn't have time to focus on her own needs. Preoccupied with her other responsibilities, she wasn't concerned when she found a small lump in her breast while showering. She mentioned it to her mother, who insisted that she see the doctor.

Anne's doctor assured her that the lump was not cancer. She was too young at the age of thirty-one and did not have a family history. Always an advocate for her daughter, her mom pushed for a biopsy.

"My surgeon was convinced that it was not cancer. I asked for a biopsy only to ease my mom's mind so that she could focus on my dad's treatment. It was such a beautiful fall day that I almost drove away from the hospital the morning of the biopsy."

Anne's decision to move forward with that biopsy changed her life. The surgeon delivered the news to her family before Anne came out of the recovery room.

"As I started to wake up from surgery, I saw a lot of friends and family in my room. I knew something was wrong. Later that afternoon the doctor came in to tell me that I had breast cancer. I remember thinking that I was in a dark hole, all alone. I wasn't educated about the disease so I was at the mercy of the doctors at that point."

Wasting no time, Anne had a radical mastectomy the next day. The doctors removed all of her lymph nodes, none of which contained cancer. It was a difficult surgery, both physically and emotionally. She was inpatient for almost two weeks, which was the standard of care after a mastectomy forty-one years ago.

"I woke up with bandages everywhere. I had no idea if I had a nipple or any resemblance of a breast. I couldn't move my arm at all. The day after surgery was the worst for me. I wanted to see the incision but had no idea what to expect. It was hard emotionally."

Anne felt fortunate that her breast cancer was caught so early. Chemotherapy was a new treatment option at the time, so her doctor did not recommend it. She was sent home to recover and worked hard to get her range of motion back by playing ball with her boys and doing her exercises with them.

"I made a decision in the hospital to be honest with my boys. I wanted to let them know I was okay and going to be okay in the long run. It took me about six weeks to bounce back and then I was back to watching the boys play ball year round and coaching girls' softball. My boys grew up thinking it was not that big of a deal that their mom was a breast cancer survivor and I'm glad that I took that approach with them."

Anne wanted to help other women with their journey so she volunteered with Reach to Recovery, offered by the American Cancer Society.

"I never felt like less of a woman because of my mastectomy. What bothered me was the isolation. Breast cancer was so secretive forty-one years ago and support was not visible. I was the youngest Reach to Recovery volunteer in the area so I traveled all over various counties. I offered support, information, and exercises to women in the hospital. Most importantly, I assured them that they would be okay and offered them hope. They had no idea that they were giving me hope and purpose, which helped me recover."

Anne also began speaking to surgeons and many groups about her experience with breast cancer. Once her youngest son left for college in 1985, she was offered a unique opportunity to work with a company that makes breast prostheses.

"I started with a group of people who are still with the company today. We are all so dedicated to the company and the cause. The CEO is from Germany and was the first person to introduce a silicone breast form to the United States. My journey with this company has been unbelievable."

Life often takes us on unexpected twists and turns, which was true for Anne, as well. After many years of marriage, Anne and her husband divorced. Being single with only one breast was quite an experience.

"I never let the fact that I'd had a mastectomy slow me down. I was always very open once the relationship deepened and if it became an issue, then I knew that person wasn't right for me anyway."

She had no idea that her true love in life was someone that she had known since her early teens. Fate reunited the old friends.

"In 1996, I became reacquainted with a man that I knew from high school. Eric had recently moved back to town so we all got together to reminisce about old times. One thing led to another and we started dating. I was nervous to tell him about my surgery because I felt like he was 'the one.' It turns out, he already knew and it was not a problem for him. We've been married for nineteen wonderful years. He supports my work and has never made me feel like less of a woman."

Anne's little boys are all grown up now and she is a stepmother to three boys from Eric's first marriage. She loves spoiling her three grandchildren and the family remains very close. Last year, one of her sons gave her the surprise of a lifetime.

"I had always loved *The Price is Right*. My son heard about a show where the studio audience would be filled with breast cancer survivors. He managed to get us tickets to go on the show. It was so much fun!"

Anne's worldwide travels include visits to China, Italy, and France. She was honored to be asked to join a group of oncologists to South America where they worked with breast cancer survivors in one of the worst areas in Columbia.

"I was afraid to go because it was so dangerous but it was one of the most amazing adventures of my life. I spent five days helping women with prostheses. Their faces were so sad but they were transformed with mastectomy bras, prostheses, and wigs. They were literally transformed before my eyes. It was the highlight of my recovery years!"

Anne recently retired after more than thirty years in the breast care industry. But she is still very involved with her mastectomy company.

"Being open about my diagnosis helped me recover. I will always be involved in some way. I can't close the door on helping other women."

Her most recent adventure was a Breast Cancer Thriver's Cruise to Belize and Mexico with two hundred breast cancer survivors and their caretakers.

"Eric gave me the cruise for our anniversary. He really wanted me to go and I was so excited to room with my friend and fellow survivor, Eunice. We've been friends for many years and we had the best time together."

Anne has celebrated the anniversary of her diagnosis every year for the last forty-one years with special dinners and cards. She looks forward to many more of those celebrations in the future.

Reflecting back on her life, she believes that she has survived breast cancer for more than four decades for many reasons.

"I had radical surgery and all of my lymph nodes removed. I was healthy and stayed active and very busy with my family and work. I believe that a good attitude helps with recovery. I try to keep stress to a minimum and remember that I can't control everything. We have to let go and focus on the moment. I am grateful for every day and I can't ask for more than that. I thank God every day for giving me the time I've had and blessing me with so much."

Looking to the future, Anne looks forward to spending more time with her three grandchildren and traveling with her husband now that they are both retired.

"My husband wanted to take me sky diving for my seventieth birthday but I said 'no thanks.' I look forward to seeing new places and maybe spending winters in Florida where it's warm. Mostly, I just want to enjoy every day."

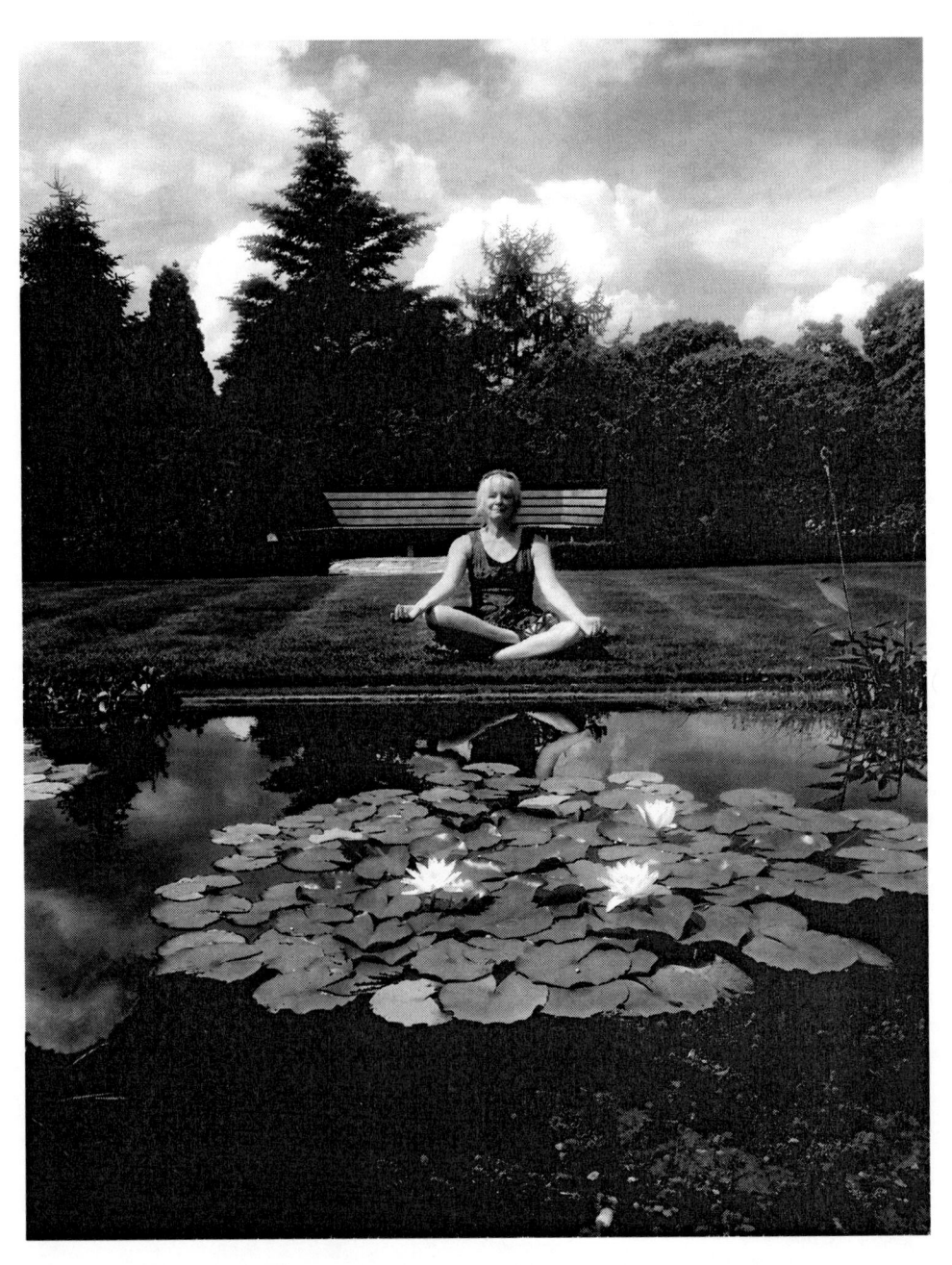

Nancy celebrating life after breast cancer with a yoga pose in Holland!

CHAPTER 2 | Nancy Bruning

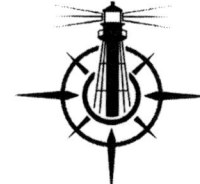

Celebrating Life Since She Was Diagnosed
in October 1980
Manhattan, NY

"I encourage women to get a second opinion, listen to everyone's advice, and then do everything you can to make the right choice for you."

Newly in love, Nancy was enjoying a successful writing career in New York. Breast cancer was never on her radar, especially at the age of thirty-one, so she wasn't overly concerned when she discovered a lump in her breast while showering. Her gynecologist was unable to detect the lump, so she told her to wait a couple of months. The lump began to grow quickly in addition to swelling in her underarm, so her gynecologist referred her to a breast surgeon.

"He tried to aspirate the lump unsuccessfully but there was no real concern. I was young and did not have a family history. He did a biopsy and then later told me that I had 'a little bit of cancer.' Everyone was shocked."

Nancy's doctor informed her that she needed a mastectomy and asked her to sign a form. Still in shock, she initially refused to sign the form. After reconsidering her options, she conceded and had a unilateral mastectomy the next day.

"I woke up after the mastectomy and had a view of the sunrise. I was deep in thought and began to cry at the beauty of that sunrise. I knew that I didn't want to die. I loved my life, my man, my career. Life was too good to leave."

Nancy spent five days in the hospital recovering from the mastectomy. Anticipating a positive pathology report, everyone was stunned with more difficult news.

"They removed seventeen lymph nodes and four of them had breast cancer cells. It wasn't a 'little bit of cancer' as they had first predicted. The tumor was 4.5 centimeters which meant that I was Stage III. I think I was in denial at the time. No one really talked about breast cancer back then and I was so young."

Nancy started a nine-month regimen of chemotherapy. The nausea was minimal and she decided against taking an anti-emetic because she felt she was taking enough drugs already. She found that she was able to minimize the nausea by eating little snacks throughout the day in addition to swimming.

"I was a freelance writer, so I was flexible with my schedule. I found a great oncologist who was holistic, so we found nutritional supplements that helped with fatigue. I stayed active throughout my chemotherapy and did hypnosis to help with anxiety."

Losing her hair was difficult at first but her mom was with her to offer support and encouragement.

"It was Thanksgiving and my hair started falling out on the way back from the beach. I tried combing it but half of it fell out in the shower. It was devastating at the time, but once it all fell out, I found a curly Shirley Temple wig. I got to be someone that I never would have been able to be with that wig. I encourage other women to have fun with their wigs. It's so much easier to get ready in the morning without hair."

After chemotherapy, Nancy had reconstruction and her journey through treatment was complete. She found it very difficult to be alone after having been monitored so closely for nearly a year.

"I was so used to chemotherapy appointments and seeing my doctor. He shook my hand and said see you in three months. I kept thinking, now what?"

Ready to move on with life, Nancy delved into a new career path. She had been incredibly frustrated throughout her journey by the lack of research available about chemotherapy. So, she decided to remedy the problem for both herself and her fellow patients.

"I wrote a book called *Coping with Chemotherapy* based on interviews with patients and professionals. I was very driven to write the book but it was hard doing those interviews because I had to relive my chemotherapy experiences. It was worth it, because I knew I would be helping others which made the whole experience meaningful for me."

Once her book about chemotherapy was written, Nancy began writing about science and health. Her career path had taken an amazing twist but this was not the only area of her life that was impacted by breast cancer.

"I found a new appreciation for every moment in life. I made the decision to minimize the things I didn't like and find more pleasure in my life."

Nancy's husband-to-be was there every step of the way through treatment. They got married and worked hard to move past her diagnosis. Her mom was very supportive but Nancy found herself yearning to meet her dad's side of the family.

"I had never known anything about my dad's side of the family and I was very motivated to meet them. I applied to a radio show in Holland to look for my family. I found my half-sister in England on the radio show live. I was stunned to learn that my other half-sister had passed away from breast cancer."

Now a survivor for more than three decades, Nancy shares her advice for women who are facing a breast cancer diagnosis.

"I encourage women to get a second opinion, listen to everyone's advice, and then do everything you can to make the right choice for you. Find an oncologist that you like, because you will have a long relationship through the years. Find someone you click with because there will be ups and downs in your journey."

Reflecting on her thoughts as to why she survived Stage III breast cancer for thirty-five years and counting, Nancy admits that initially, she did not believe she would be a long-term survivor.

"I just did my best. I put one foot in front of the other and kept on going. I try to treat myself well and do something kind every day, which has been good for me. I eat a healthy diet, exercise, and take supplements, all of which keep me healthy."

Nancy is still writing, but she also gets paid to teach exercise classes in the park.

"I get to go outside and be in nature. I want others to go out in nature and move their bodies, living life to the fullest. I challenge people with the question, 'You moved your body, but did you move your soul?' It's important to know the difference."

Looking to the future, Nancy plans to enjoy life with her family and friends. Her bucket list is diverse and has changed since her experience with breast cancer.

"I fulfilled one of my bucket list items during chemotherapy. I had always wanted to learn to play a musical instrument, so I took lessons, learning to play the recorder and read musical notes. Now, I have a big desire to help others. My goal is to create groups all over the country that offer exercise outside in the park."

You can learn more about Nancy's exercise groups by visiting www.nancercize.net.

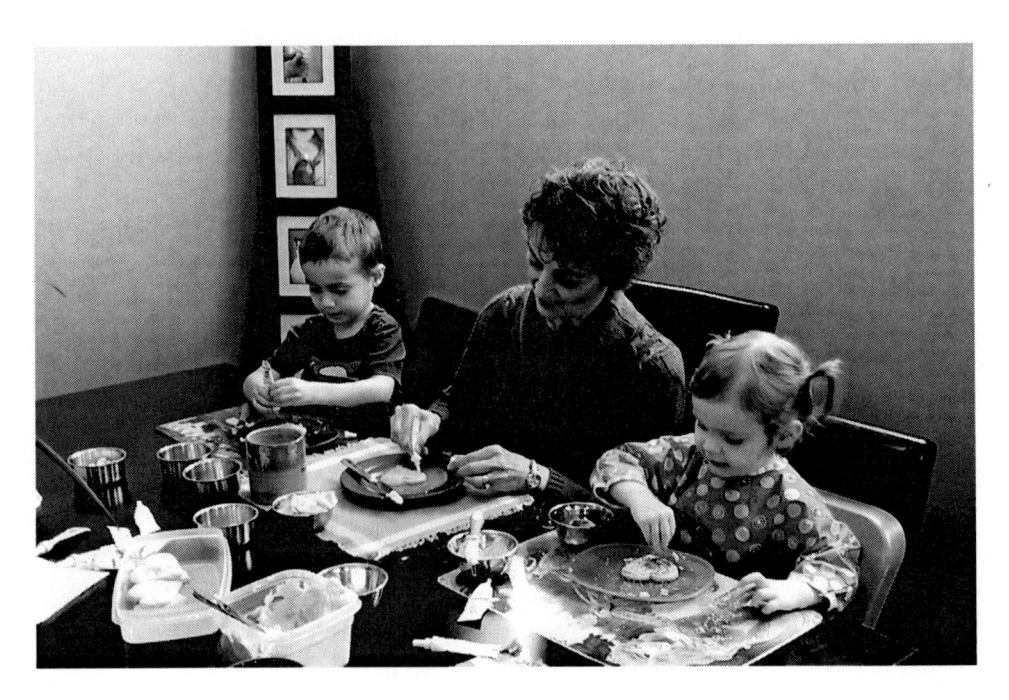

Barbara celebrating life after breast cancer with her grandchildren, Wesley and Kira!

Chapter 3
Barbara Cunnings-Versaevel

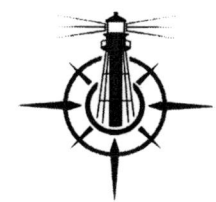

Celebrating Life Since She Was Diagnosed
in Fall 1990
Calgary, Alberta Canada

"Breast cancer gave me back myself."

A former professional dancer, Barbara had an active lifestyle and stayed busy with her husband and fourteen-year-old son. Her days of traveling extensively with her dancing career were behind her, but she still enjoyed walking, jogging, and Tai Chi. One random day, she was doing pushups when she felt a tightness at the top of her breast. Further investigation led her to discover a small lump the size of a pea. She called her doctor immediately.

"The lump did not show up on the mammogram but I could feel it. My doctor told me to come back in six months. I went back six months later and the lump had grown to 2.5 centimeters. I could tell from the doctor's face during the biopsy that it was cancer."

Barbara's suspicions were confirmed. She had breast cancer. She underwent a lumpectomy and lymph node dissection. The pathology report indicated that fourteen out of twenty-two lymph nodes were involved. She was diagnosed with Stage III triple-negative breast cancer. Minimal research supported her doctor's frightening information about the aggressiveness of triple-negative breast cancer.

"I drew into myself a bit when I was diagnosed. I did a lot of walking, researching, and journaling to get through the initial fear. I started researching long-term breast cancer survivors and felt that I could become a long-term survivor if I made changes in my life."

Barbara's doctors prescribed intense chemotherapy. She shared a hospital room with a wonderful woman and quickly bonded with her new "cancer buddy." The support she received from her friend helped them both through the dark days of treatment.

"The side effects of chemotherapy were brutal. I had been so active my entire life but it would take four days after each treatment before I could even go for a good walk. Things were very different twenty-five years ago."

Back then, Barbara's treatment plan included three chemotherapy treatments followed by radiation then three more chemotherapy treatments. She stayed as active as possible by walking, doing Tai Chi, and meditation when her body was strong enough for physical activity. Once treatment was over, she reevaluated her entire life which led her to make to a very difficult decision.

"Surviving breast cancer gave me back myself. I was in a bad situation in my personal life and I knew that I had to make changes if I wanted to live long enough to be there to watch my son become a man. I decided to leave a bad marriage and start from ground zero. Once I left, I learned who I was and reclaimed myself."

Barbara set out on a quest to become educated in all aspects of her life with the goal of preventing a recurrence.

"I began researching complementary medicine. I found that a combination of traditional medicine, complementary medicine, energy, diet, and supplements all work together to access what is inside of us to heal. Healing is hard work but it is rewarding because it's about living a wonderful life."

Once Barbara implemented her findings into her own life, she felt compelled to teach other women how to reduce their risk. Her passion to help others grew when she learned that most cancer survivors could not afford complementary medicine as it was not covered by insurance. She began networking with like-minded advocates, determined to make a difference. She partnered with two other people to start Wellspring Calgary. It is a unique program that provides emotional, psychological, and practical support to cancer patients. Programs include group classes, expressive therapies, energy work, and educational workshops.

"Wellspring offers all of the tools that cancer survivors need to help themselves through any kind of cancer. We offer services to the patient, their families, and caregivers all free of charge. It's a healing journey supported by fundraising. Our vision is that 'No one has to face cancer alone.'"

Barbara facilitates two programs, including one of the passions that she had given up as a young wife and mother.

"I've come full circle. I am dancing again and I teach dance at Wellspring. I'm also writing. I'm strong in me again. My sense of life is great because my work fulfills me."

Twenty-five years have passed since Barbara was diagnosed with breast cancer. Her little boy is an adult now. He is married and has blessed her with two amazing grandchildren and an awesome daughter-in-law. Barbara has learned to find balance in her life between work and maintaining her healthy lifestyle.

"I get a monthly massage, meditate, and stay very active. I learned to say 'no' more often, which is hard to do. Breast cancer does not define me and I no longer focus on being a survivor. I focus on staying healthy."

After recovering from a difficult first marriage and discovering inner happiness, Barbara met a wonderful man. They recently celebrated their fifteenth wedding anniversary.

Reflecting back on her life, Barbara shares her insight as to why she believes she has survived breast cancer for more than two decades and counting.

"I think it's a combination of things. Part of it is my purpose in life with the job that I've been given to do. I have a strong faith and a one-on-one relationship with God. I am always aware of the need for balance in my life and I try to avoid stress. I have developed a lot of tools to stay on a safe, healthy path in my life."

Looking to the future, Barbara is excited to start traveling more extensively.

"One of the perks of being a professional dancer was the travel. I'm taking a leap of faith by traveling to a small village in the South of France. I'm renting a house for a month so I can live there, experience life, and write about it. It's the first of many times that I will do this, as I love to travel. I walk to the beat of a different drummer and not everyone understands that, but it works for me."

You can learn more about Wellspring Calgary by visiting www.wellspringcalgary.com.

Learn more about Barbara's travel adventures and follow The Cancer Help Hub online by visiting www.cancerhelphub.com.

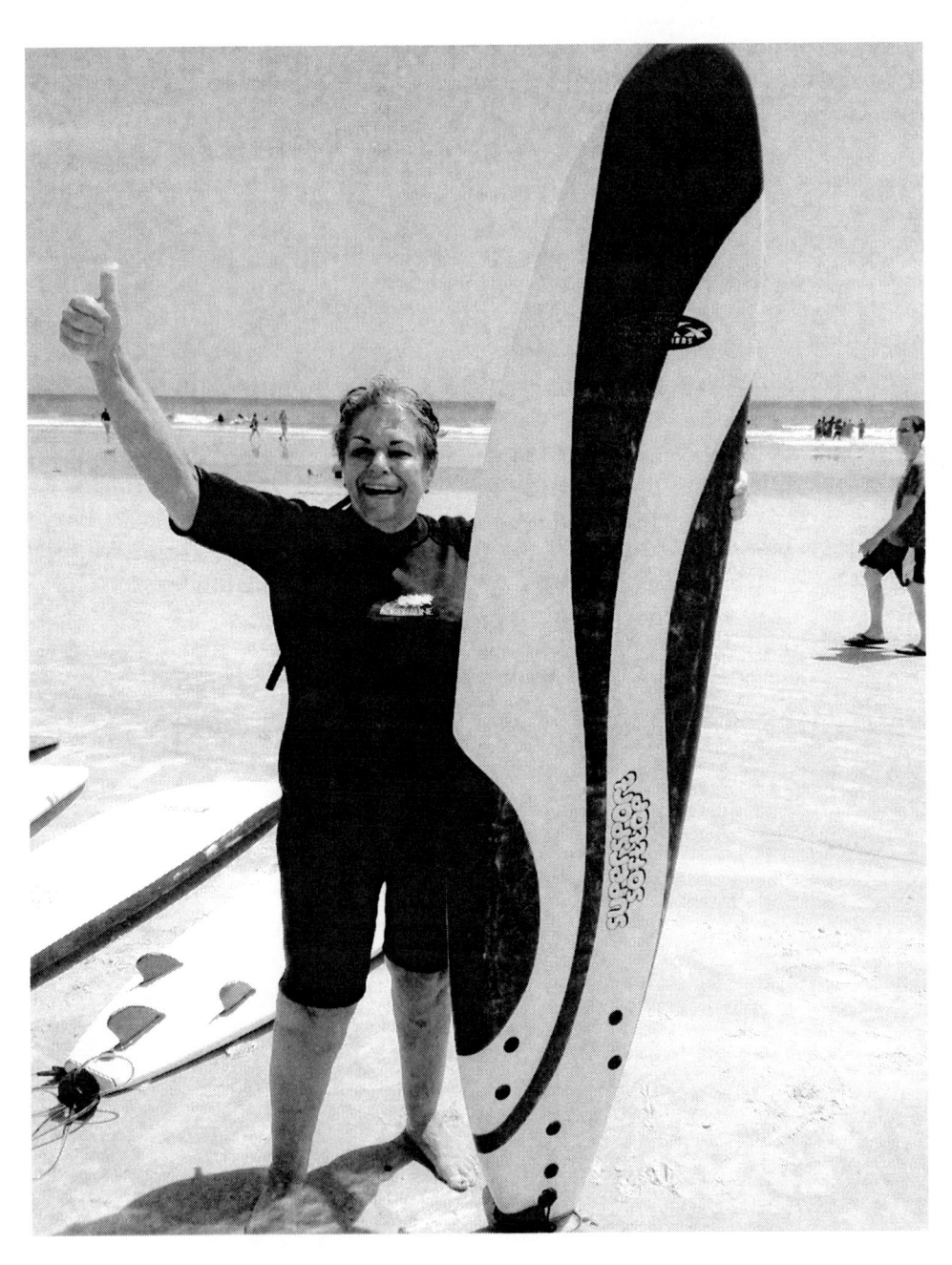

Bobbi celebrating life after breast cancer by learning to surf!

CHAPTER 4
Bobbi de Cordova-Hanks

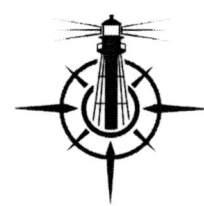

Celebrating Life Since She Was Diagnosed
in May 1986
Jacksonville, FL

"Who knew that a bass-playing Brooklyn babe could become an advocate, speaking in front of Congress? Breast cancer has truly been a gift for me."

Life was full of adventure and travel for Bobbi. Her twenty-five-year career as a professional bass player and singer was full of fun and excitement but something new had entered the forefront of Bobbi's world. She met her soul mate, Jerry! They married and relocated to a new city when Bobbi noticed a problem with her breasts.

"I was resting on my stomach after a fierce tennis match with my husband. I woke up and my breasts felt like they had turned to stone. I told Jerry that a foreign object had lodged itself into my breasts."

Breast health had been vital for Bobbi after having a lump removed in her early thirties. Keenly aware of her fibrocystic breast tissue, she had been visiting her gynecologist for a clinical exam every six months for many years.

"I had been fighting fatigue but my doctor told me it was early menopause. I knew something was wrong when he did the exam. He sent me to an oncologist and scheduled my first mammogram at the age of fifty."

The mammogram was followed by a surgical biopsy. The pathology report confirmed everyone's worst fears. Bobbi had breast cancer.

"It was such a shock. I had just gotten married to a man who had lost his first wife to misdiagnosed ovarian cancer. How could I put Jerry through this again? I knew I was in for the fight of my life."

Surgery was the first step in Bobbi's treatment journey. The surgeon recommended a mastectomy and removal of all of her lymph nodes. Still recovering from surgery, Bobbi was devastated to learn the results of her pathology report.

"The tumor was large at six centimeters and had invaded lymph nodes. He told me that I had Stage IIIB breast cancer and only had five years to live. I was so angry with him. There is only one person who knows when my time is up."

Bobbi's sense of humor and positive outlook carried her through a year of chemotherapy. She continued to play tennis throughout her treatment. There were dark days but she had lots of support from her family and friends.

"I had relatives come out of the woodwork to support me. The toughest part was the lack of resources. I wanted to learn about the diagnosis and treatment but this was before the time of the Internet. There weren't many advocacy groups so I had to wing it and rely on my doctors."

Breast cancer treatment was not the only obstacle Bobbi was facing at the time.

"The company that I was working for found out about my diagnosis. They were so sure I was going to die that they closed down and literally chained the doors shut to avoid the insurance premiums from my treatment. I found myself with a cancer diagnosis, no job, and no insurance."

Well qualified, Bobbi began her job search and was the number-one candidate for several jobs but wasn't being hired. She discovered the truth from a local headhunter that she had been working with to find a job.

"This was before laws were passed to prevent discrimination against medical issues. The companies were able to run a report with my social security number and determine that I was a breast cancer survivor so they wouldn't hire me. It was tragic."

Once treatment ended, Bobbi lost her security blanket of actively fighting breast cancer. She went to work for a community college and came up with a new idea.

"There weren't any support groups in the entire city, so I asked the president at the college if I could utilize a classroom setting to start one. He challenged me to write a curriculum and syllabus and that's how we started Bosom Buddies."

Bosom Buddies is a support group offered free of charge to women with a breast cancer diagnosis. The organization has served more than seven thousand women over the last twenty-six years. She retired from the college in 1999 and spends all of her time running Bosom Buddies, in addition to serving on many boards related to breast cancer.

"My job with Bosom Buddies is twenty-four/seven with very little money but that's not what it's about. I remember feeling isolated after my diagnosis and I never want anyone to have that experience. We match women with buddies by age, marital status, common interests, and neighborhoods. We are a zany group of women who have formed lifelong friendships while living beyond breast cancer. We also educate women about their rights throughout their treatment process. There is so much love shared among all of us."

As she continued to work with Bosom Buddies, Bobbi realized that there was a significant need for information about life after breast cancer.

"I became very active with a national organization that works to ensure the rights of survivors. I have served on the board and presented at numerous conferences throughout the nation. Who knew that a bass-playing Brooklyn babe could become an advocate, speaking in front of Congress? Breast cancer has truly been a gift for me."

Breast cancer has not been the only challenge that Bobbi has faced over the years. She was diagnosed with metastatic thyroid cancer in 1999. Her treatment was incredibly intense but successful. Once again, Bobbi's doctors were astounded. In December of 2012, she was very sick with problems in her colon. Her doctors told her that it wasn't looking good and planned an invasive surgery that would create the need for a colostomy bag, if she survived the surgery.

"I started singing and crying. I lit a candle and asked God for one more miracle. I went back in for one last set of scans before surgery and the doctor walked in with the results. My colon had healed itself. My doctor sent me home without surgery. I went home and fell on my knees. God knows that my women in Bosom Buddies need me."

Most recently, Bobbi was diagnosed with skin cancer in 2014. In her younger years, she spent five years living on a boat, which increased her risk, as well as her exposure to the Florida sun. She took the diagnosis in stride and had a successful surgery to remove the cancer.

Throughout the years, Bobbi's husband, Jerry, has been instrumental in her recovery from her multiple cancer diagnoses.

"When someone is diagnosed, it becomes everyone's cancer. The invisible survivor is the caregiver and they need support but are often overlooked. Jerry and I wrote a book together called *Tears of Joy* which talks about my journey through cancer and his experiences as a caregiver. We talk to groups all over the country and in Canada about our experiences. We share laughter and tears and have a lot of fun meeting new people."

Bobbi has talked to thousands of women since her diagnosis and offers her advice for moving past a cancer diagnosis.

"Being in limbo is so hard. You get diagnosed and you're not sure how to go on living. Many women live in fear of dying. I tell them to get their house in order and make plans in the event the cancer comes back or treatment doesn't work. Then stop worrying about dying and go on with life."

Breast cancer changed Bobbi's entire life in so many ways. In addition to starting Bosom Buddies and becoming an advocate for cancer survivorship, she went back to performing but for a much different audience.

"I had a spiritual awakening which was totally due to breast cancer. I was born Jewish but married an Episcopalian. I felt like I had a hole in my heart and soul so one day, I went to church with my husband. The next weekend, I was singing in the choir and was later baptized."

Reflecting back over nearly three decades since her breast cancer diagnosis, Bobbi has several thoughts as to why she has survived for so long and is still going strong.

"My doctors have no idea why I'm still alive. They consider me a miracle. I tell everyone that I'm too busy to die. It's not in my Day-Timer and no other woman will wear my jewelry. Somehow, it's worked. God has a purpose for me and my women need me."

Looking to the future, Bobbi plans to continue working with Bosom Buddies for many years to come. She joined forces with The Women's Center of Jacksonville, as part of its community education department, to ensure that her mission with her beloved organization will go on indefinitely. She plans to travel with her husband and continue advocating for her fellow cancer survivors. She also has one other hope for the future.

"My years as a professional bass player/singer ruined my hearing. A year of chemo and eight years of Tamoxifen finished it off. I would love to get the bass in my hands and hear the music again."

You can learn more about Bosom Buddies and Bobbi's book, Tears of Joy, *by visiting www.speakersforlife.com.*

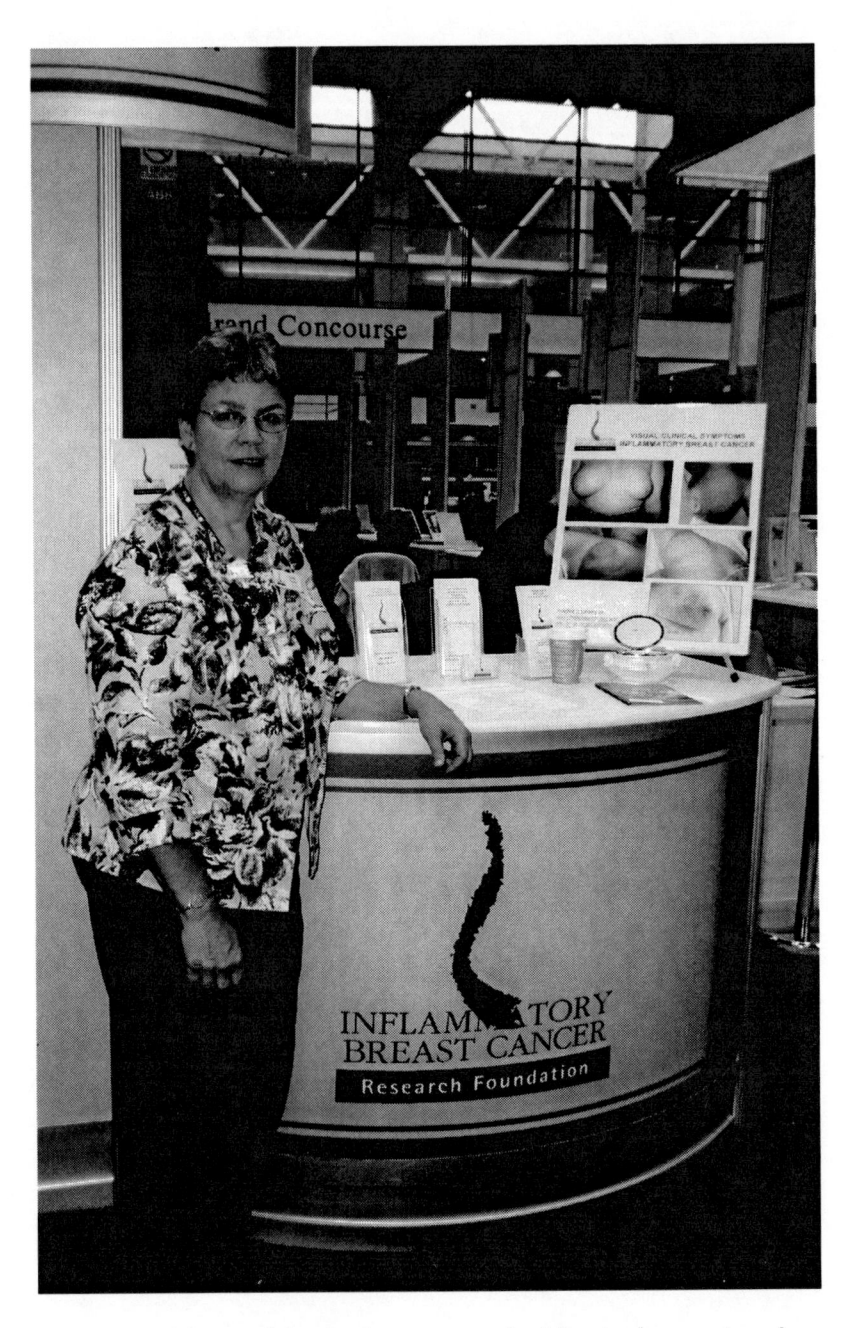

Ginny celebrating life after breast cancer by following her passion of educating others about inflammatory breast cancer.

Chapter 5 | Ginny Mason

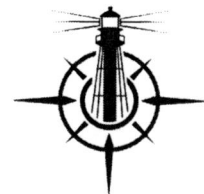

Celebrating Life Since She Was Diagnosed
in March 1994
West Lafayette, Indiana

"I wasn't sure how much longer I would survive, so I wrote a letter to my granddaughter. Twenty years later, I handed her that letter just days before her wedding. It was such a gift to be there throughout her life."

A preacher's wife, mother to a senior in high school, and an outpatient mental health nurse.... Ginny was busy! Perhaps her most exciting new role in life was as grandmother to a baby girl. She lived a healthy, active lifestyle and had a goal for the future: she wanted to become a certified nurse midwife.

At the age of forty, she was experiencing hormone fluctuations so she wasn't overly concerned when one of her breasts had occasional shooting pain and seemed swollen.

"I didn't have a palpable lump but the symptoms kept getting worse. One day, I was getting out of the shower and my husband told me that my breast looked sick. It had indentations and was swollen so we went to see my doctor, who also happened to be a family friend."

The doctor sent her for a mammogram which showed dense breast tissue and perhaps a cyst. Out of character for a quiet preacher's wife, Ginny asked to speak to the radiologist.

"He said the mammogram was fine and asked me, 'What's the problem?' I told him that my breast looked funny and asked him to look at it. He said I was a hypochondriac nurse and told me to go home. I went home and looked up breast cysts which were common at my age so I tried to ignore the problem for the next three months."

When the pain became intolerable, Ginny went back to see her doctor/family friend. After unsuccessfully attempting to aspirate a thickened area, he recommended a biopsy.

"I had a biopsy in his office with no anesthesia. By then, the pain had been so intense for so long that I was fine with ice for numbing. I dropped off the sample at the lab on my way back to my office. I didn't have a family history of cancer and I didn't have a lump, so cancer never even crossed my mind."

She met with her doctor the next day in a large conference room.

"His face was flat and he took my hand. I thought, 'This can't be good.' He told me that I had inflammatory breast cancer. On a scale of one to ten, this is not the one you want. He told me that he had an oncologist waiting downstairs to start my chemotherapy. He walked me down to the oncology unit and the doctors were staring at me like I was a dead man walking."

The meeting with the oncologist was overwhelming. After discussing the details of her cancer, he recommended starting chemotherapy immediately.

"I realized what they were telling me and told them that I couldn't call my husband and tell him to come get me, I've had chemotherapy. He didn't even know I had breast cancer. I told them that this had been brewing for months and that we could wait until Monday to start treatment. I think they were afraid I would walk out and not come back."

Ginny went back to work like nothing happened. She kept her secret from her daughter, who came by to drop off Ginny's granddaughter. She was determined to discuss her news with her husband first.

"At four p.m., I told my supervisor that I needed Monday afternoon off for a medical appointment. He said he hoped it was nothing serious. So I told him the diagnosis and that I was given twelve to eighteen months to live and he started to cry. He hugged me and told me that he would do anything I needed. If I wanted to work that would be fine but if I didn't want to work, he would hold my job. He was great throughout all of it."

Ginny drove home in a rainstorm, rehearsing what she would say to her husband. The words didn't come out exactly as she planned.

"I blurted out, 'I have breast cancer and I'm going to die.' We cried together, hugged each other, and cried some more. When we were all cried out, we were sitting there in silence. The storm outside stopped and a huge rainbow filled the sky. We could see both ends of it and I had a sense of peace come over me. Even if I didn't survive, I knew everything would be okay."

Inflammatory breast cancer is uncommon and aggressive. Ginny's oncologist presented her case to the National Cancer Institute tumor board which recommended neo-adjuvant chemotherapy (chemotherapy before surgery) which was a new idea at that time.

She worked throughout her six months of chemotherapy, taking off one afternoon every two to three weeks for her treatments. She was very open with her diagnosis with everyone she encountered which resulted in support and prayers throughout treatment.

Once chemotherapy was complete, Ginny had a modified radical unilateral mastectomy. The surgery was extensive requiring a week-long stay in the hospital due to some complications.

"I was still in the hospital when the surgeon tearfully told me that I had so much residual disease after chemotherapy that his original prognosis of twelve to eighteen months was optimistic. He told me to get my affairs in order. The cancer was in eleven of the sixteen lymph nodes removed. Not only did I have inflammatory breast cancer, but I also had invasive ductal carcinoma and mucinous carcinoma which is very rare. I went back to my belief that I cannot control what happens to me, only how I respond. I could either decide to die and let my body catch up to my mind or I could live every day to the fullest."

Ginny went home to recover, taking off two weeks and two days from work which was well below what her doctors recommended. The best therapy was rocking her baby granddaughter. Radiation was the next step in her treatment plan followed by Tamoxifen. She stayed busy and focused on enjoying life.

"When I made it to a year after my diagnosis, I thought, 'Ha ha folks! I'm still here.' But I wasn't sure how much longer I would survive, so I wrote a letter to each of my loved ones, even my granddaughter. I knew that I probably wouldn't be around to see her grow up. I wrote those letters in March 1995. Twenty years later, I handed my granddaughter her letter just days before her wedding, which was the same week as the anniversary of my diagnosis. I was an emotional wreck at her wedding rehearsal. It was such a gift to be there and watch her grow up and then at her wedding. I have been given so many years that no one expected."

Ginny's journey through breast cancer changed her entire life. After treatment, she worked full time while obtaining a bachelor's degree in nursing. She started a support group in her community for breast cancer survivors and felt the need to do more for women with inflammatory breast cancer (IBC).

"I was doing research on the Internet when I connected with a man in Alaska who had lost his wife to inflammatory breast cancer. He was preparing to start an organization focused on research and awareness of IBC. We met with him in 1999 on a trip to Alaska to celebrate the five-year anniversary of my diagnosis and my graduation from college. I was excited about the idea of an organization dedicated to the research of IBC. That was the start of the Inflammatory Breast Cancer Research Foundation and I have been very involved since its beginning. We celebrated fifteen years as an organization in August 2014."

Ginny became the executive director of the foundation in 2003 and later the president. The primary focus is to facilitate research for inflammatory breast cancer through grants and collaboration, in addition to advocating for patients and offering patient support. The website is extensive, offering information for patients and the medical community as well as a telephone help line.

"Yes, breast cancer is in my past but this foundation isn't about me. I needed to be a voice and give back. I represent the voice of the patient population and the women who died at a young age from this disease. There is real satisfaction at the end of the day knowing that we are helping others."

Ginny's diligence with the Inflammatory Breast Cancer Research Foundation has changed the way doctors are instructed to view skin changes to the breasts. It has also changed the way inflammatory breast cancer is treated through involvement with the National Comprehensive Cancer Network (NCCN) guideline panels.

"Inflammatory breast cancer is not a garden variety breast cancer. Before 2008, women with this disease were being treated with the same guidelines as locally advanced breast cancer which included a lumpectomy and radiation. We worked for three years to implement treatment guidelines specific to inflammatory breast cancer. There is not a lot of instant gratification but we have helped make big changes in the scheme of things."

She has spoken to groups throughout the world about IBC and met some of the women whose lives were saved as a result of her dedication. A monthly email newsletter published by the foundation offers education and hope to patients and doctors coping with the disease.

"I met a woman in 2003 who had been diagnosed with IBC. She had decided not to do any treatment because she thought she was going to die. I was already nine years out from my diagnosis which gave her enough hope to do chemotherapy. She wrote an article for our newsletter recently, sharing her story as a ten-year survivor."

Ginny is relentless in her quest to educate others about IBC and to find a cure. It has become her passion in life. She always has educational brochures and bookmarks in her purse.

"I have come a long way since that quiet minister's wife in 1994. People say that I am like a dripping faucet, annoying but persistent. I will work as an advocate for IBC until we have it all figured out or until I can't do it physically."

Ginny wears a pin from the foundation depicting a tumor cell cluster that often prompts questions from strangers.

"I tell them that my pin represents inflammatory breast cancer that tried to kill me then educate them about it. My message is simple. If you have any changes in your breasts that don't go away within two weeks, see your doctor for an evaluation and don't take no for an answer. A lump is not required to have breast cancer. I'll never know the ripple effect of our work but everyone who is educated becomes a volunteer. They may save a life with that information."

Ginny served on the Oncologic Drug Advisory Board for the Food and Drug Administration (FDA) for four years. It was a challenging but educational experience.

"It was hard because we had to review all types of oncology drugs, not just for breast cancer. But I learned the drug approval process which made me a better advocate."

Reflecting on the more than twenty-one years since her diagnosis, Ginny shares her insight as to why she has survived this particularly aggressive form of breast cancer.

"I really don't know. A lot of people ask me that question. I love vegetables and I love to walk but I still enjoy an occasional diet pop and chocolate. Some say that God wasn't finished with me yet. I don't say that out of respect for the women who haven't survived, I don't want to assume God was finished with them. However, I do feel as though I have a responsibility to use the time I have been given to help others. Faith has been an incredible part of it all. I do believe that while being positive may not lengthen your life it can help you live a better life while you are here."

Ginny's husband has been incredibly supportive throughout their entire marriage. Her daughter has blessed them with a total of ten grandchildren!

"Part of my dedication to breast cancer research in general relates to my seven granddaughters. I don't want them to have to worry about breast cancer, especially since my daughter was diagnosed with early stage, aggressive breast cancer at the age of twenty-seven."

Looking to the future, Ginny plans to continue her work with the Inflammatory Breast Cancer Research Foundation as long as she is able. She would love to travel to visit family in Europe and perhaps move closer to her daughter's family after her husband retires.

"I would love to be closer to watch them grow up. I want them to know me so we Skype a lot and we make special memories when we are all together."

She recently checked an item off of her bucket list this year while on a business trip.

"I went to see a Broadway play while in New York City. I have always wanted to go and it was awesome! I love the music to *Phantom of the Opera* and had a hard time not singing along."

For more information about the Inflammatory Breast Cancer Research Foundation, please visit www.ibcresearch.org.

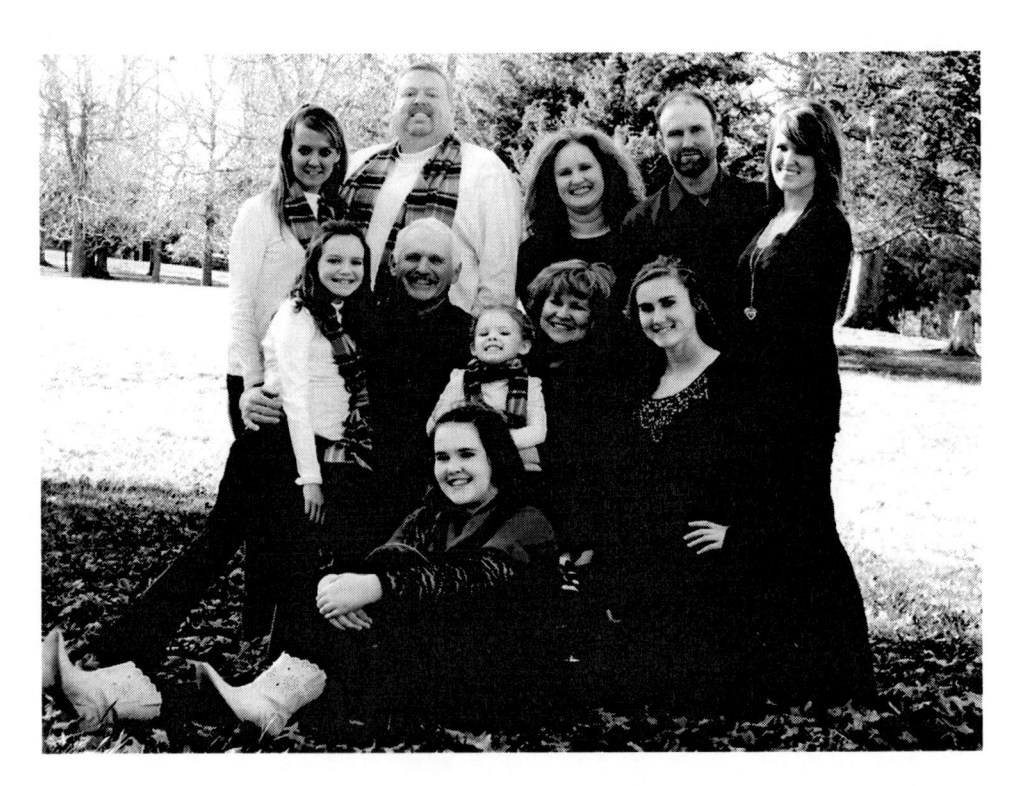

Beverly celebrating life after breast cancer with her beautiful family!

CHAPTER 6 | Beverly Vote

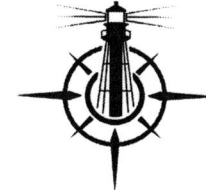

Celebrating Life Since She Was Diagnosed
in August 1992
Lebanon, MO

*"Surviving is our starting point.
Thriving is our original design"*

Beverly was living her version of the iconic American Dream in 1992. Happily married with two children, she had spent many years building her award-winning insurance agency in the small town of Lebanon, Missouri. Active in her community, involved in her children's lives, and dedicated to both her marriage and her career, she worked hard to be happy and have the things that she thought would bring her joy and satisfaction. Unbeknownst to her at the time, her diagnosis would be the catalyst for transforming her perspective about the deeper meaning of her life.

"I was just about to take a shower when I intuitively felt my right breast and found a walnut-sized lump. Before the day was out, I called my gynecologist to make an appointment. Over the course of a year, I was misdiagnosed four times. Today I understand part of the misdiagnosis was because I had dense breast tissue. Even though I had to push my doctor to have a mammogram and further diagnostic testing, I didn't fully understand the meaning of being my own health advocate at the time."

A needle biopsy confirmed what Beverly had suspected all along. She had breast cancer.

"In the flash of being diagnosed with Stage III breast cancer, I went from being an executive decision maker for my clients to being so overwhelmed and confused that I couldn't even order off a menu. How was I to have any confidence making a life-saving decision if I couldn't even decide between chicken or fish? Especially when my doctor for more than twenty years blew off my own health needs? The experience of being diagnosed with breast cancer taught me how easy it is for fear to take over our minds, our common sense and one's faith."

Beverly's treatment plan included a mastectomy and six months of chemotherapy. Two years after her first diagnosis, she was advised that she had three small lumps in her other breast. The words from her oncology and medical teams came back to haunt her.

"My first prognosis was bleak. My doctors repeatedly told me it was highly probable that the cancer would come back and it would be aggressive and deadly when it returned. I felt I had very few resources. This was before the Internet and was at a time when everyone I knew who had been diagnosed with cancer died shortly after their diagnosis."

With yet another short and intense learning curve before her, Beverly leaned heavily on her faith.

"I experienced God's outreach to me. There were many life-changing moments in my journey that I will never forget and I remain grateful to this day. These moments taught me that God is always present and our most challenging experiences can teach us something. It taught me that we are more than a body and that we each have something on a core level to heal in our life."

Beverly spent years as an avid student of mind-body concepts, wondering why she healed and others didn't and trying to overcome survivor's guilt. She was internally obsessed about her true purpose of her life.

No longer a part of the executive world, Beverly's life moved in another new direction one sunny morning in the privacy of her sunroom. She had been contemplating purchasing a local magazine that was struggling. Using a yellow pad, she was weighing the pros and cons of the purchase and what it would take to make the publication work.

"The focus of the magazine shifted when I heard a voice in the sunroom. I was all alone, yet I heard the voice clearly. I answered the voice and agreed to the voice that the magazine would be about breast cancer."

From that moment forward, Beverly became focused and energized on publishing a magazine about breast cancer. It was during that moment of clarity that she envisioned the title *Breast Cancer Wellness Magazine*, which would have a national and global reach.

"I believe it was no accident that I was connected with a woman in sales and marketing. Suddenly we had three weeks before going to print with the first issue of the magazine. In the sunroom once again, I sat in the middle of the floor on my knees in prayer and told God if He was willing to show up for this, then I was too. In that very sacred moment, I felt a calm and peace come over me. Through the experience of publishing the magazine, I continue to learn about a higher power and purpose in each of our lives."

Beverly has spent much of her life after breast cancer inspiring others. She has interviewed hundreds of survivors, experts, and celebrities for the breast cancer wellness mission which has not only inspired her readers, but continues to be a catalyst for growth in her own life.

Reflecting back on the twenty-three years since her diagnosis, Beverly shares her insight into why she has survived breast cancer for more than two decades and is still loving life.

"Breast cancer helped me to see things more from a soul level and less from an ego perspective. I experience a great satisfaction from helping others. I continue to learn from others who have walked the path before me. Too often, women do not even know what brings them joy and this is a sad realization that we have chosen to let the busyness of life and other people's agendas rob from us what is most important."

Always open to learning, Beverly has enjoyed spending time with several experts in the field of mind-body concepts.

"Dr. Bernie Siegel taught me that a healing journey begins by healing one's life. It took me several months to internalize this concept and now I encourage women to break free from their greatest fears about their life and to believe in themselves even when they feel no one else understands."

Recognizing that there are many challenges of healing from breast cancer and the need for positive support, Beverly started the annual Breast Cancer Thrivers Cruise in 2005. Hosted by the magazine, the cruise is unlike any other. Breast cancer survivors from around the world come together to share positive support, laughter, learning, and inspiration while enjoying the luxury of a cruise.

"I love hosting the cruises! I began the annual event because I wanted to celebrate life with others. On the cruise, we celebrate each other and make lasting friendships."

Beverly has already fulfilled one important item on her bucket list.

"There was a time that I didn't believe I would be alive to see my first granddaughter start kindergarten. When Lindsey graduated from high school, I couldn't contain my sobs of gratitude that day. She went on and graduated with honors from college. I now have five granddaughters and I continue to enjoy all of their special milestones."

Beverly plans to continue fulfilling her life mission to help change the culture and consciousness about breast cancer through her work with *Breast Cancer Wellness Magazine*, by hosting the Breast Cancer Thrivers Cruises, hosting special retreats, and with an upcoming book about the mind-body connection and how it relates to breast cancer. On a personal level, she also plans to continue enjoying her family and spending time on the lake with David, her husband for more than forty years.

Learn more about Beverly's magazine and the Breast Cancer Thrivers Cruise by visiting www.breastcancerwellness.com.

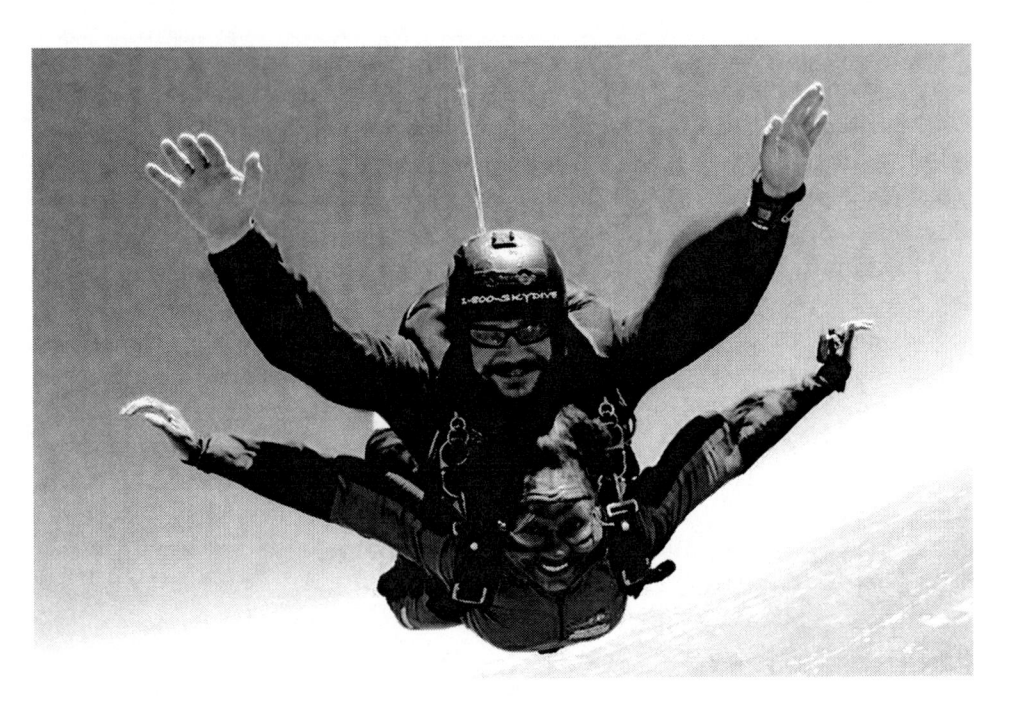

Karen celebrating life after breast cancer by skydiving for her sixtieth birthday!

CHAPTER 7
Karen Eubanks Jackson

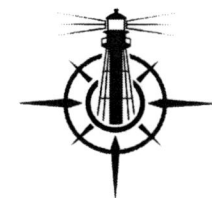

Celebrating Life Since She Was Diagnosed
in October 1993
Houston, TX

"I didn't think it was awesome to start Sisters Network Inc., I just thought it was necessary. The breast cancer survival statistics are grim for African Americans, but knowledge is power. I followed my vision of a network of African American women across the nation . . . and that was my focus."

Karen Jackson was no stranger to breast cancer. Determined to be proactive after losing her aunt to the disease, she had her first mammogram at age thirty-five. Her doctors were not concerned when a mammogram revealed a palatable mass because she was so young. Like so many other women, Karen had an instinctual feeling that something was not right, so she asked for further testing.

"I knew something was wrong with my breast. I insisted that they do an ultrasound and they finally humored me. My physician shed a tear and told me he was so sorry when it turned out to be breast cancer. I was devastated to learn about my diagnosis even though I had done everything right."

A lumpectomy confirmed that Karen had Stage II breast cancer. While she did not have lymph node involvement, her cancer was 3.5 centimeters, high grade. Her doctors prescribed six months of chemotherapy and six weeks of radiation and offered a grim prognosis.

"They told me that I only had five years to live. I wanted to spend those years near my daughter who was getting ready to start a family, so I relocated to Houston, Texas. I started looking for a national support organization for African American women."

Karen was disappointed to learn that no such national organization existed. Worse yet, many of her family and friends refused to discuss breast cancer. Determined to make the most of the last five years of her life, Karen had a vision of a network of African American women across the nation.

"I seldom pay attention to what others say. My mother raised me to think for myself, which saved my life when I insisted on an early mammogram. I saw a need and I had a vision so I started working on my vision in the middle of chemotherapy."

The side effects of treatment were difficult for Karen but she knew that she was fighting for her life. The fatigue was challenging but she kept herself busy by drawing up plans for the new organization and by journaling. Her husband, Kyle, was there to support her every step of the way along with her daughter, Caleen, which helped her move forward.

"I came from a family of community-minded people so I didn't think it was awesome to start Sisters Network, I just thought it was necessary. The breast cancer survival statistics are grim for African Americans but knowledge is power. I followed my vision of a network of African American women across the nation that would offer education and support about breast cancer and that was my focus."

Karen started Sisters Network Inc. in 1994 with the goal of stopping the silence and shame of breast cancer that prevents many African American women from obtaining proper preventative care. This shame makes early detection less likely and lowers survival rates. She kept busy with the organization throughout her cancer treatment. It continued to grow and flourish, expanding from one state to another.

Karen struggled with lymphedema as a result of treatment but overall remained healthy as the years passed. She celebrated her five-year mark and then stopped counting. She was focused on making a difference for her sisters throughout the nation. Today, Sisters Network Inc. is in forty-three cities in twenty-two states. She now has a staff of seven to help her run the organization with more than three thousand members and associate members nationwide.

"I never want to have to say that we can't help someone. It has been a labor of love and the longer that I have been involved, there is even more to do."

Sisters Network Inc. takes much of Karen's time but she has been instrumental in creating other programs for the organization, as well. The Gift of Life Block Walk began in 1995. This unique program brings women together to knock on doors, educate others about breast cancer, schedule mammograms, and invite them to the community center for health screenings.

"In this day and age, people still don't know the facts about breast cancer. We are determined to stop the silence. Many women are afraid that if they talk about it, they will get it. We save lives through this program then they in turn save more lives by sharing their experience."

Karen has spent the last twenty years advocating for African American women in the fight against breast cancer. She received difficult news in early 2014: a new occurrence of breast cancer.

"I feel blessed because it was DCIS (ductal carcinoma in situ). This time, I found it early because of my knowledge. I was prepared for any future problems. If my toe hurts, I see my oncologist first, which is why we found it early. Every woman needs knowledge to find their breast cancer at this stage."

Karen recently launched another new program called Teens 4 Pink. The goal is to empower teens ages twelve to sixteen to talk to blood relatives about breast cancer. This simple act will change the paradigm within families. The teens attend a training and earn the title of "Pink Ambassador." Teens 4 Pink is designed for the African American population but will become a universal program for all cultures in the near future. As a national organization, they were fortunate to receive funding from a major pharmaceutical company.

"I'm very proud of this program which was inspired by my granddaughters. They are very aware of the mission and the importance of education about breast cancer. We are changing the next generation."

As Karen reflects on more than two decades since her breast cancer diagnosis, she shares her insight on surviving this disease for so long.

"I believe that being optimistic about life in general has something to do with it. I always try to find the good in what's happening which helps with health in general. We all have challenges but we can't solve them all at once. Deal with them one at a time so you won't get overwhelmed."

Karen also credits her faith for carrying her through her diagnosis and for setting her life on a new course so many years ago in the midst of chemotherapy.

"Faith brought Sisters Network to me. It took me awhile to accept this. I was chosen to do this. It was not on my list of things to do with my life. I was driven to do it. My talent is that I can organize others and that's exactly what I've done. I'm proud to see that so many women are being impacted by my efforts."

Karen leads by example with the many programs that she has developed, speaking and traveling internationally, and helping promote legislation on the state and federal level. She has served on The International Breast Cancer Research Foundation, Center for Research on Minority Health, CARRA, S.P.I.R.I.T., and the American Society of Breast Disease.

In her free time, she enjoys her busy life with her loving, devoted husband Kyle, who has supported Karen's endeavors throughout the years. She lives close to her daughter, Caleen, and her granddaughters, Brianna and Alexis.

Karen loves adventure and has lived out her dream of riding in a hot air balloon and skydiving. She also has other adventures planned for the future.

You can learn more about all of Karen's programs by visiting www.sistersnetworkinc.org.

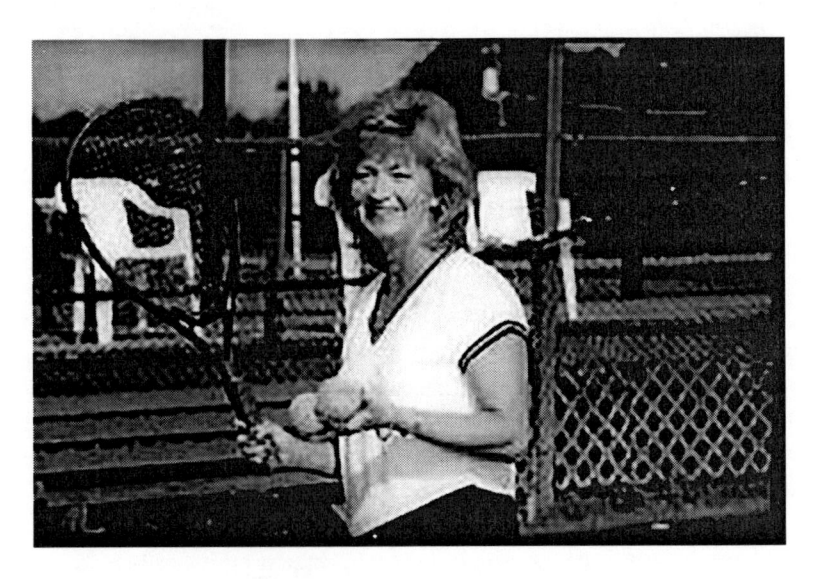

*Eunice celebrating life decades after breast cancer
by enjoying a fierce game of tennis!*

CHAPTER 8 | Eunice Walker

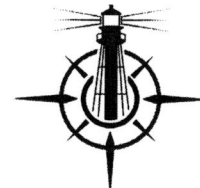

Celebrating Life Since She Was Diagnosed
in November 1987
Huntsville, AL

"We have to believe in our recovery. I firmly believe that survival is a privilege but recovery is a choice."

Full of spunk and tenacity, Eunice had experienced much loss by the age of forty. Her older sister and two brothers had recently passed away and her eighteen-year-old son lost his life in a tragic car accident.

"We were still recovering from the death of my son but we were starting to enjoy life again. I was staying busy and extremely active with tennis. Life was starting to move in a positive direction when a mammogram detected a lump in my breast."

Eunice had been down this road before. At the age of twenty-six, the fear of having discovered a lump in her breast was replaced with relief when a biopsy confirmed that it was benign. She had practiced vigilant breast health since that time, with mammograms every six months and monthly self-exams. She followed her instincts after the mammogram discovered this second lump.

"At first they thought it was calcification. I had to wait three weeks for the pathology report. Nine different pathologists in Atlanta looked at the tumor then they sent it to St. Louis. Deep down, I knew it was breast cancer."

Eunice's instincts were correct. The final pathology report indicated that breast cancer was detected underneath the calcifications. Her initial reaction was fear.

"I was terrified, just like everyone else who is diagnosed. I had lost my older sister to breast cancer. My sons were fifteen and sixteen and had gone through enough loss. I wanted to be there for them. Then, I thought about the traumas that I had overcome. I asked God for His strength which helped me put everything into perspective."

Once the initial shock wore off, Eunice weighed her surgery options carefully.

"I had a gut feeling that I wanted a mastectomy, even though I had been given the option of a lumpectomy with radiation. I knew that I could survive without a breast. I never felt like less of a woman because of my decision."

Eunice's doctor recommended that she wait for a year to have reconstruction. He also suggested a prophylactic mastectomy on the other side but advised her to hold off on the second surgery for at least one year. She felt fortunate when she learned that she would not need chemotherapy or radiation.

"My sister had cobalt treatments and she had a rough time. She fought for four years and she didn't make it. I didn't have a battle with breast cancer. My battle was recovering the use of my arm after complications from plastic surgery."

Eunice scheduled her prophylactic mastectomy with immediate reconstruction one year after her initial surgery. Unfortunately, she experienced significant complications. She had a tear in her chest wall muscle. The implant was removed and the doctor shared difficult news. She had a brachial plexus injury due to overstretching her arms during surgery.

"The doctors told me that there was little chance of regaining movement in that arm and I knew if it remained paralyzed, I would never play tennis again. I was determined to prove them wrong."

Eunice spent a month in the hospital participating in intense physical and occupational therapy. As the nerves slowly regenerated, the paralysis was replaced with severe pain. She left the hospital with many months of work ahead but she eventually regained the use of her arm, hand, and fingers.

"It was my tenaciousness and sheer determination to play tennis again that helped me through the hardest days. I gained back ninety percent usage of my arm and hand. I developed a mean two-handed forehand tennis swing and I played tennis for many years. Don't ever tell me I can't . . . I will show you that I can. We have to believe in our recovery. I firmly believe that survival is a privilege but recovery is a choice."

Eunice's mantra and determination led her to create her business, Special Touch by Eunice, a mastectomy and wig boutique. The first three years she worked out of her home.

"There was such a need for a mastectomy boutique in my area. I had to go behind a little curtain in a health food store for my fitting. It was degrading but it sparked an idea. Six years after my diagnosis, I started my business with the support of my family. It has grown so much through the years and we have a great reputation. We offer pre- and post-surgery consultation and carry great products."

Doctors from nearby cities and states refer their patients to Eunice's business. Women drive from miles around based on word of mouth and they always return when they need more supplies. The atmosphere is warm and reassuring for women facing such a difficult time in life. Eunice has a small staff, all of whom are breast cancer survivors. They offer hugs of support, in addition to education and supplies.

"Every day I pray to God to bless me greatly and make me a blessing to someone today. He has given me a ministry and a purpose for my life and I try to fulfill it every day with my business. It fills my need to be a counselor because I offer a lot of emotional support to my ladies."

Although Eunice had significant problems with her reconstruction surgery, she is supportive of women making the right choice for them.

"When women come into my office, I tell them that I couldn't feel like more of a woman. If they want reconstruction for their head, I will support them and offer to help them find the right medical team. But there are so many great prostheses out there that can help you look great and feel confident. It's a personal choice."

The boutique has kept her going throughout the years. Her sons have been supportive through it all. They are all grown up now and live within close proximity of Eunice.

"My boys are awesome. They had a band at one point and they still play together on occasion. One son and his wife are both artists and the other son is engaged to a wonderful woman. I love my boys and enjoy spending time with them."

Breast cancer shaped Eunice's career, but it also changed her life in unexpected ways.

"I became more confident after breast cancer. It changed my life in a positive way. I knew I could do anything I wanted to do if I left it in the Lord's hands. It took the first fifty years of my life to discover why I'm here. I figured God would give me another fifty years to do what He wants me to do."

Reflecting back on her life, Eunice shares her insight as to why she has survived breast cancer for nearly three decades and counting.

"It was early detection that saved me. We caught my breast cancer so early because they watched me like a hawk after my sister was diagnosed. I am blessed every day. God is good. He gave me the strength to get through it and put wonderful people in my life when I needed them. I'm forever grateful and I know how fortunate I am to have survived breast cancer for twenty-eight years. I have a lot to be thankful for."

Eunice recently enjoyed a Breast Cancer Thrivers Cruise with her longtime friend and fellow survivor, Anne. They were accompanied by nearly two hundred other breast cancer survivors in the Caribbean. She had a great time and hopes to go on an Alaskan cruise in years to come.

Looking to the future, Eunice plans to write a book based on recovering from the loss of her son and her experience with having a paralyzed arm. She is contemplating retirement sometime soon.

"I would love to go somewhere by myself to a remote area with my laptop by a beach or a lake and chill out. It would be my time with God and the beautiful world."

Learn more about Eunice's mastectomy boutique by visiting www.specialtouchbyeunice.com.

Celebrating Life Decades After Breast Cancer

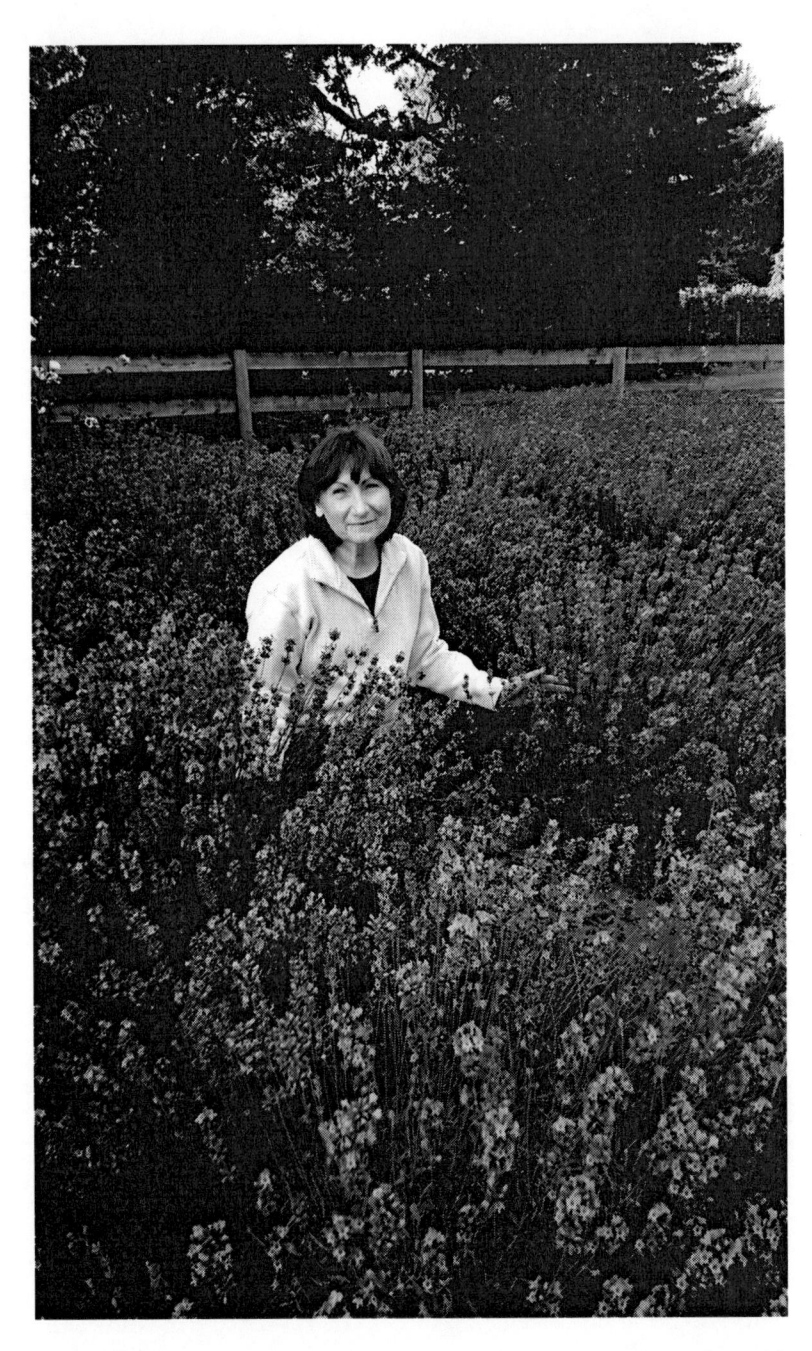

Chris celebrating life after breast cancer in the midst of her lavender fields!

CHAPTER 9 | Chris Mulder

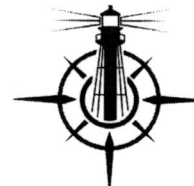

Celebrating Life Since She Was Diagnosed
in June 1986
Wilsonville, OR

"I have spent many years of my life helping others through all stages of breast cancer. I tell women to take one day at a time. Educate yourself and find the support you need to keep moving forward with hope."

The Barn Owl Nursery is a picturesque herb and lavender farm located in Oregon, stretching over five acres. Christine (Chris) started her peaceful, home-based retail herb farm with her husband, Ed, in 1982. Tending to her nursery business, her first "baby," Chris found peace and comfort in her garden, especially after a miscarriage. Determined to start a family, she decided to visit her doctor for a checkup.

"I had a history of lumps in my breasts for several years, but they came and went with my cycle. I never worried about them. I was young and did not have a history of breast cancer. But one of the lumps had changed so I went to see the doctor to have it checked before trying for another baby."

A proactive doctor, years ahead of her time, ordered Chris's first mammogram at the age of thirty-four. A mammogram at that age was almost unheard of at the time, but Chris credits that imaging with saving her life.

The results of mammogram dictated bilateral biopsies. The lump she was worried about was benign, but the biopsy of the calcifications in her other breast revealed low-grade DCIS (ductal carcinoma in situ). Chris was offered the option of a lumpectomy with radiation or a modified radical mastectomy. She wanted to be aggressive with treatment, so she opted for a mastectomy on the side with breast cancer. After reviewing the pathology report with her surgeon, and getting another opinion, she decided to have a simple mastectomy on the other side six weeks later.

"Some members of my family wondered why I would 'give up' a healthy breast, but I was steadfast in my decision. I wanted to start a family and be around to raise my children. I felt that having a prophylactic mastectomy would give me peace of mind."

Delayed reconstruction began four months after the second mastectomy and it was a positive step for Chris. The results did not meet her high expectations, but her new breasts gave her confidence and she felt like she could move on with her life. But as so many women have discovered, life after breast cancer can be more challenging than expected.

"I realized that I needed to mourn the loss of my breasts before moving on. I joined two different breast cancer support groups. There were not many groups being offered in my community and I had to go outside of my hospital to find them."

As Chris healed over the next two years, she contemplated starting a family. At that time, there was very little research about how pregnancy might impact breast cancer survivors. After becoming informed with the limited information available, she made a monumental decision in her life. She would not have children. Once this decision was made, she decided to change her career path.

"Deciding not to have children was a difficult decision, harder than my treatment decision for breast cancer. It changed my entire life plan. I was already putting my energy into helping develop a breast cancer support group and establishing a breast cancer lending library for patients at the hospital where I was treated. I was determined to educate myself and provide support to try to help other women diagnosed with breast cancer in my community."

With the help of an oncology nurse, her surgeons, and a social worker, they combined two types of support groups into one. It consisted of an eight-week course designed to educate and comfort women coping with a breast cancer diagnosis. She quickly realized that the women attending the support group needed a one-on-one approach before their treatment. She continued to help with an ongoing support group, while she developed her second "baby," the only Breast Cancer Outreach Program in her area.

Breast cancer changed everything for Chris, but her new career choices have helped countless women through the Breast Cancer Outreach Program (BCOP), that she coordinated for twenty-five years through the support of Providence Cancer Center. The support groups, patient libraries, and the BCOP continue to offer invaluable information to patients, their families and people in the community who want to learn more about breast cancer.

"The women I have met inspire me with their strength and courage, even though some have not survived. They taught me that we all deal with breast cancer in our own way, in our own time."

As her confidence in working with the community grew, she served on a committee with two other breast cancer survivors to help bring the Komen Race for the Cure to Portland, Oregon, her third "baby." She took on the job as education chair for the Portland/SW Washington Komen affiliate. In 1996, she chaired a planning committee to develop the first Breast Cancer Issues Conference held in Portland.

"I have spent a good part of my life supporting patients through all stages of breast cancer. I tell women to take one day at a time. Educate yourself by using the many resources that are available to help you make informed decisions. Find the support you need to get you through each day, and keep moving forward with hope."

While Chris's many contributions to the breast cancer community have been appreciated and respected, the services of the Breast Cancer Outreach Program volunteers are still the heart of all the resources she helped develop. The BCOP is perhaps best known for the comfort pillows that volunteers make to give to newly diagnosed patients after their surgery.

"We recognized the need for pillows early on. We call them comfort pillows and offer them for support after surgery. We have collected donated materials and volunteers take the time to sew them and add their personal touches. Many patients that have received these pillows hang onto them long after they have healed from their breast cancer treatment."

Looking back over the last twenty nine years since her diagnosis, Chris shares her insight as to why she has survived the disease for nearly three decades.

"My early detection and attitude helped me survive and cope with life after my diagnosis. I chose to become involved with helping others and became healthier with diet and exercise. I also learned to recognize stress and reevaluate the need for balance in my life."

Breast cancer changed Chris's entire life path and those changes have been positive in her life.

"I wouldn't go as far as to say that I am grateful for my breast cancer diagnosis, but I am grateful for the many positive outcomes that came from that diagnosis as a result. My relationship with my husband deepened, I gained more confidence to work with the community, and I have a deeper appreciation for life."

Chris recently retired as coordinator of the BCOP, but she continues to volunteer for the outreach program that she developed so many years ago. She has been enjoying long hours tending to her first "baby," her herb nursery and lavender farm. She is currently serving as President of the Oregon Lavender Association and helping to sponsor a NW Regional Lavender Conference in Portland for lavender farmers across the nation. Looking to the future, she plans to travel and spend more time with family and friends. Her most anticipated future plan is a road trip to Alaska with her husband.

For more information about Chris's lavender farm, please visit www.barnowlnursery.com.

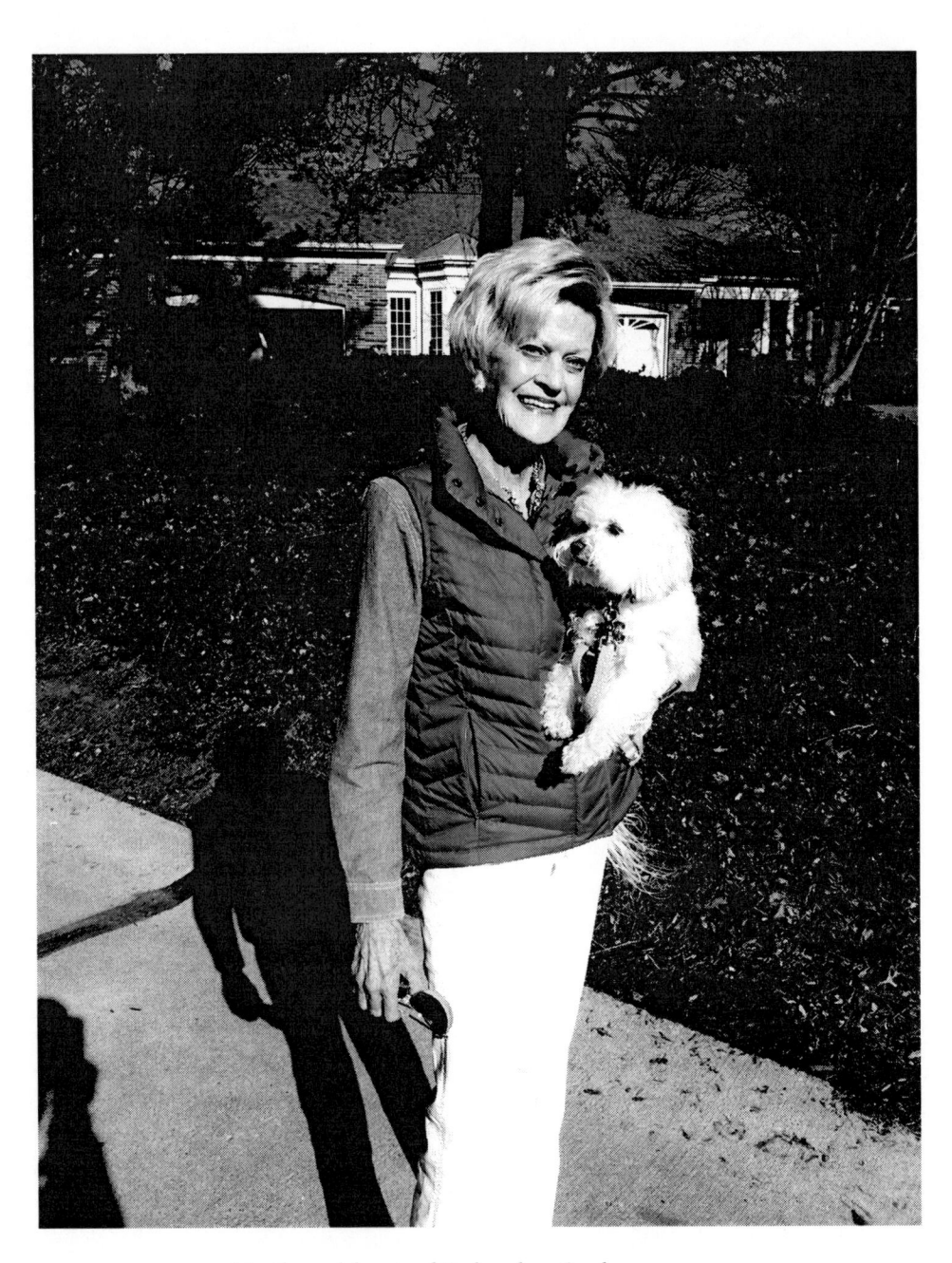

*Marilyn celebrating life decades after breast cancer
with her beloved dog, Murphy!*

Chapter 10 | Marilyn Fries

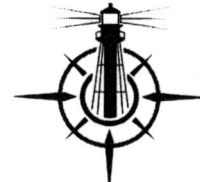

Celebrating Life Since She Was Diagnosed
in March 1983
St. Louis, MO

"I wasn't sure that I could help other women recovering from breast cancer, but I did. That was a turning point for me. That's when I stopped crying."

Happily married for many years, Marilyn was busy enjoying life with her husband and their three grown children and spoiling their grandchildren. Breast cancer was the last thing on her mind when she saw a public service message from Sophia Lauren advocating for monthly self-exams.

"I thought if Sophia Lauren can do it, so can I, even though breast cancer did not run in my family. I was shocked to find a lump that day."

Marilyn's husband was well connected in the medical community due to his role as a radiologist. He found a general surgeon who performed a needle biopsy. After waiting with bated breath, the family was relieved to learn that the lump was fibrocystic changes. She went back to life as usual until the lump returned a few months later.

This time, a surgical biopsy was performed. Once again, the lump came back as benign, but the pathology showed cancer in the tissue next to the lump. Lobular carcinoma in situ, a less-common type of cancer that often escapes detection by a mammogram until the cancer has advanced beyond the breast tissue. Marilyn's benign fibrocystic changes allowed her doctors to discover the breast cancer early, but the diagnosis was overwhelming.

"I can remember the moment so well. The surgeon told me that I had breast cancer and would need to have my breasts removed. I looked around the room to see who she was talking to, because it couldn't possibly be me. I was absolutely stunned and started to cry. I didn't stop crying for weeks and weeks."

Marilyn had caught her cancer early but her doctor warned her that lobular carcinoma is likely to have a mirror image in her other breast, hence the recommendation for a bilateral mastectomy. Disfigurement was at the forefront of Marilyn's concerns. Bilateral mastectomies were performed differently thirty-two years ago and reconstruction was very new at the time. Luckily, her husband's connections helped them research the option of reconstruction. They consulted with a surgeon and plastic surgeon which resulted in the plan to perform a modified radical bilateral mastectomy with reconstruction.

"It never occurred to me that I would die from breast cancer. I just knew how disfiguring a mastectomy could be for women and that played a huge role in my thinking. I cried a lot before and after surgery."

Marilyn healed physically but still struggled with her tears. She needed to heal mentally which led her to volunteer with Reach to Recovery offered by the American Cancer Society. She decided to dress like a "million bucks" while visiting women in the hospital who were recovering from surgery after breast cancer. The goal was to offer them hope for the future.

"I was so nervous when I got my first assignment. I got into the car and put the key into the ignition and started to cry. I wasn't sure that I could help other women recovering from breast cancer, but I did. That was a turning point for me. That's when I stopped crying."

She continues to advocate for early detection.

"I was very determined that women do self-exams monthly and mammograms every year. It is so easy to do and so important. This became my crusade."

Her fears of disfigurement long in the past, she has enjoyed a new sense of normalcy due to her implants. Having lived through decades of scares about health concerns related to implants, she has never had a problem with hers, even after thirty-one years. She often shares a very personal message with women who are concerned about disfigurement after breast cancer surgery.

"It might be hard to believe but you can look whole and beautiful again, even in a swimsuit. There are so many options with prostheses and reconstruction."

Looking back on her journey through breast cancer, Marilyn shares her insight as to why she has survived breast cancer for more than three decades.

"We caught it early and I had great doctors. Helping others helped me heal which was so important for me to move past my diagnosis.

Marilyn's life has been full of happiness and love since her diagnosis. She spent much of her life volunteering and traveling extensively with her husband. They traveled to Paris, Venice, Hong Kong, Singapore, and two walking tours in Europe, to name just a few of her amazing memories. One trip stands out among all of the rest.

"If I live to be one hundred and take more trips, it won't compare to the safari that we went on in Kenya and Tanzania. It was the most wonderful trip ever."

After a lifetime of marriage, Marilyn was able to support her husband through his diagnosis of Parkinson's and dementia until he recently passed away.

"He was a brave man and never complained. I miss him but I am surrounded by love from my three children, who all live close, my nine grandchildren and six great-grandchildren."

She plans to continue volunteering and spoiling her great-grandbabies for many years to come.

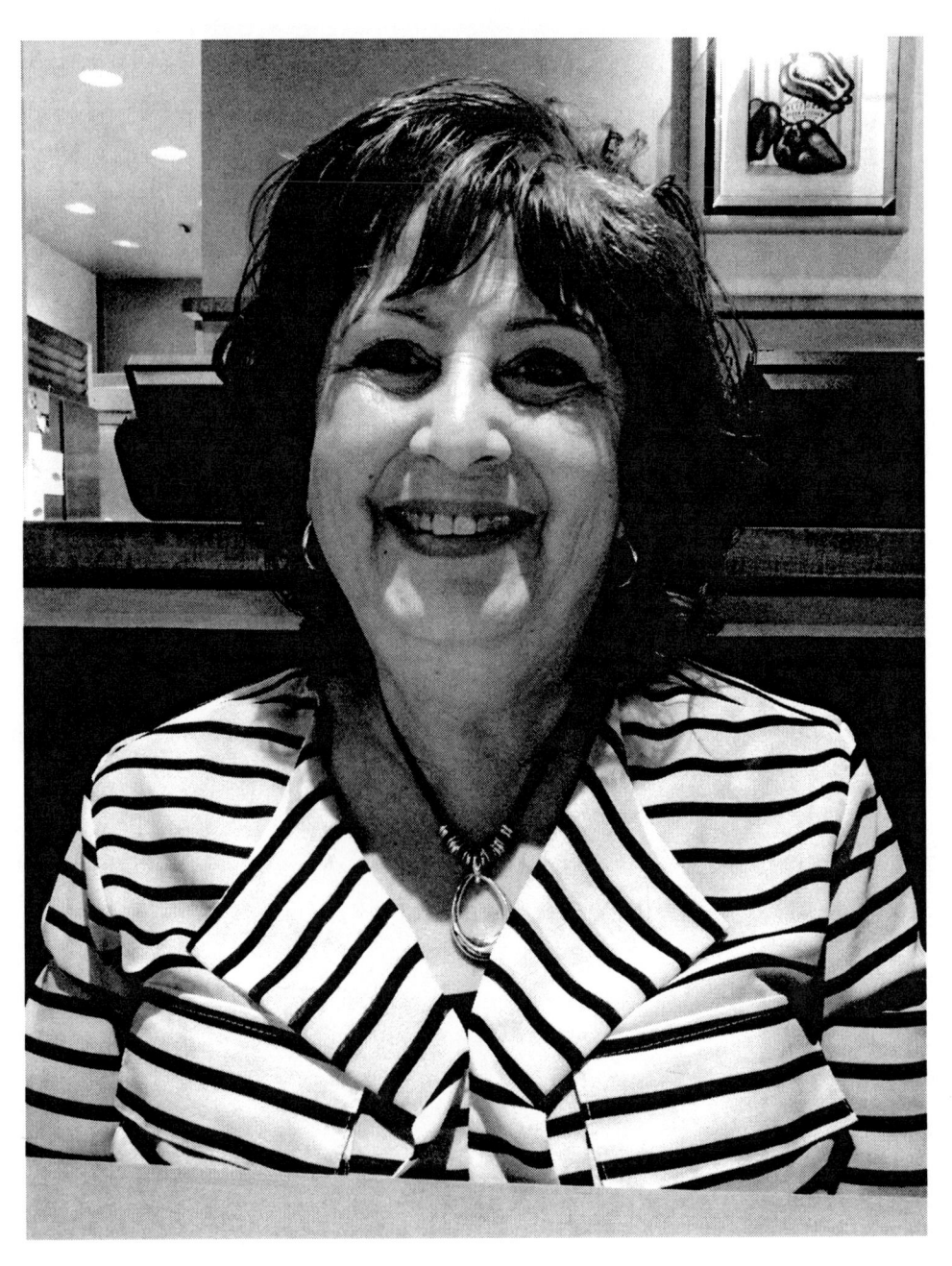

Odell celebrating life thirty-four years after breast cancer.

Chapter 11 | Odell Sauls

Celebrating Life Since She Was Diagnosed
in June 1981
Tampa, FL

"I finally felt like I was doing something worthwhile. I was helping others and following my dreams. I tell women that breast cancer happens for a purpose, not punishment."

Odell's biggest fear in life was that one day, she would be diagnosed with breast cancer and need a disfiguring radical mastectomy, like her mom. Her worst fears came true when she was only thirty-six years old with young children, ages six and fifteen.

We all have high points and low points in life. Odell was having a truly low point in her life. Her mother had recently passed away and her marriage was on rocky ground. As if that weren't enough stress, she found a lump in her breast. Her biggest fear in life had been a breast cancer diagnosis, so she postponed going to the doctor. Life was busy with her children and Odell was overwhelmed with her many responsibilities. But the lump didn't go away, prompting her to see her doctor. He referred her to a surgeon for a biopsy which resulted in the news that Odell had dreaded hearing for so long. She had breast cancer and needed a mastectomy.

"My first thought was that I was going to look like my mom. This has always been my biggest fear in life and now it was coming true. I never thought I would die from it. I cried a lot at first."

Odell was relieved when she discovered that she could have a modified radical mastectomy. This type of surgery would not leave her body as disfigured as she feared but she had to cope with other challenging news. The pathology showed that the breast cancer had spread to her lymph nodes, so chemotherapy was the next step for treatment. The plan was one year of chemotherapy, one treatment each month.

"It was yucky. I had lots of nausea and lost my hair, eyelashes, eyebrows . . . everything."

Odell was working in a doctor's office in the same building as her oncologist's office. She would go to work, then walk down the hall for her chemotherapy treatments. Nine months into her chemotherapy treatments, her marriage ended in divorce. In addition to the many side effects of chemotherapy, she had to adjust to life as a single mom.

"It was the hardest time of my life. But my friends, family, and coworkers all rallied to help me. God helped me through all of it."

Odell dealt with more life stressors simultaneously than many people face in a lifetime but she pushed through those challenges with the help of her faith, family, and friends.

"Breast cancer caused my faith to go deeper. I realized after it was all over that it wasn't the worst thing that could ever happen in life."

Faced with her own mortality, Odell decided that it was time to follow her dream in life. She had always wanted to be a nurse so after chemotherapy was finished, she enrolled in nursing school. She knew the odds of being accepted were slim, but it was time to take a chance on her dreams. She was accepted and once she graduated, she used her own experience with breast cancer to help others. She went to work as a nurse in an oncology office.

She offered support to her patients in a way that few others can but she learned from her patients as well. She educated herself on the option of reconstruction and eventually opted for this surgery to complete her journey through breast cancer treatment. Odell also started a support group for breast cancer survivors and later worked as a prosthesis fitter.

"I finally felt like I was doing something worthwhile. I was helping others and following my dreams. I tell women that breast cancer happens for a purpose, not punishment."

Odell used her sense of humor to heal and help her fellow breast cancer survivors. She couldn't contain her laughter while sharing a story about a mishap that occurred prior to her reconstruction surgery:

"I got a new prosthesis and I wanted to go swimming. I didn't have a mastectomy swimsuit so I wore a shirt over my regular swimsuit. I was having fun swimming when all of sudden, something hit me in the chin. I looked down and there was my prosthesis, floating in the water. It was hysterical and I started laughing. I tell women that it's better to laugh when these things happen."

Reflecting back over the last thirty-four years since her breast cancer diagnosis, Odell has only one answer as to why she has survived for more than three decades:

"God is the reason that I am here today. I have no other answer. I cannot imagine my life without God. I rely on Him to get me through everything."

Today, Odell has a full, busy life which centers around her family and her work. She lives near both of her adult children who were so supportive during her treatment. Her favorite pastime is spoiling her children and grandchildren, playing an active role in their lives. She continues to utilize her degree as a registered nurse, but now she helps patients over the phone. This allows her to work from home and be available to help out with the grandchildren as needed. Most recently, she is working on one of her bucket list items.

"I'm writing a book about growing up in the French Quarter. It started as a memoir but has turned into a novel. At first the book chronicles my life, starting with my birth in New Orleans and it ends with me returning to the French Quarter to open a nursery for underprivileged children to teach them about God. I'm thinking about calling it *St. Philip Street*, where my life began. I can't wait to share it with the world!"

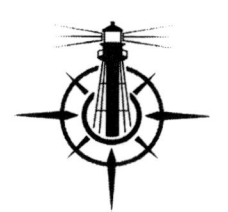

Section 2

The Power of a Positive Attitude

Breast cancer can be all consuming at times. The overwhelming barrage of oncology terms, a new world of treatment planning and outcome discussions. We're often left feeling overwhelmed and out of control. But the women in this section know that there is one thing that breast cancer cannot control. Our attitude. We have the ability to search for the rainbows through the storm of breast cancer. It isn't always easy, but even on the darkest days, the rainbows are always there, just waiting to be discovered.

While a positive attitude is not a cure for breast cancer, we can learn from these survivor stories that a positive attitude makes every day that we are alive much more fulfilling. Research has shown that a positive approach to treatment can improve a patient's response to pain, side effects, and medication.

Consider how your journey through life might change if you started searching for the rainbows through the storm. The amazing women in this chapter share their insight into the power of positive thinking and how it continues to impact their lives decades after breast cancer.

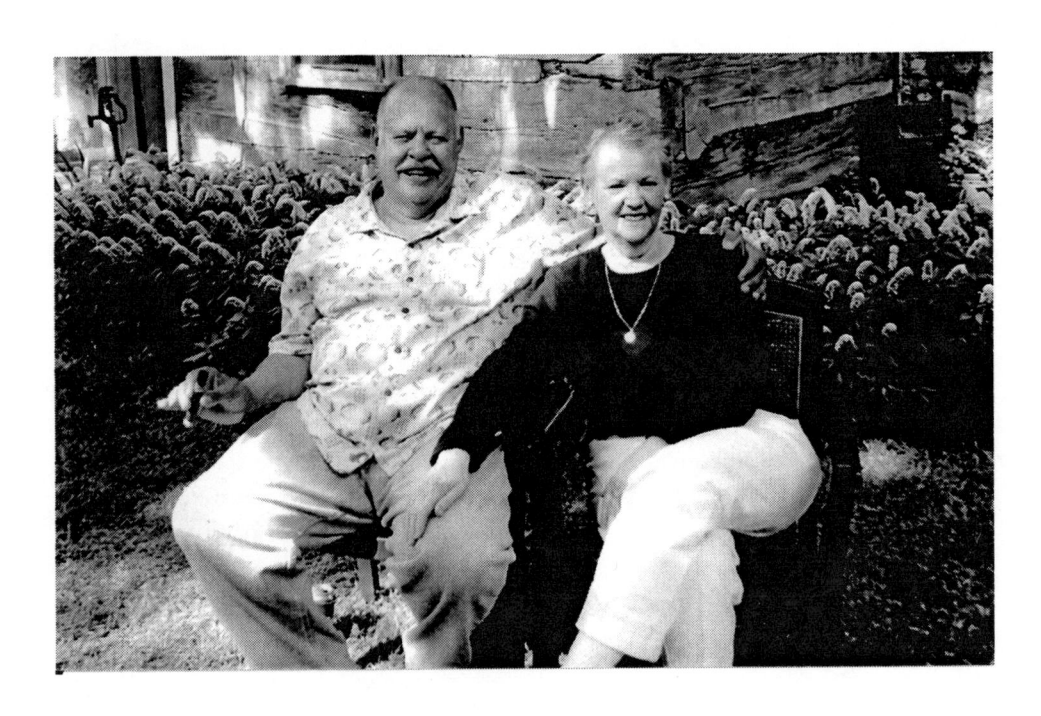

Carolyn celebrating life after breast cancer with her husband, Jim, on their fiftieth wedding anniversary.

Chapter 12 | Carolyn Smith

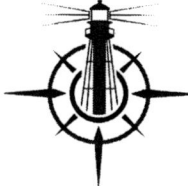

Celebrating Life Since She Was Diagnosed
in November 1965
St. Peters, MO

"I think about my journey through breast cancer on that day every year. My sisters call me to tell me they are thankful that I'm still here. I've watched my five children grow up and now they have their own families. My life has been a good one."

Fifty years ago, Carolyn was a very busy full-time mom to five young children. She gave little consideration to the brown spot in her bra until two weeks later, she discovered a similar brown spot. Breast cancer was the furthest thing from her mind. She didn't have a lump and she was only thirty years old. A trip to her doctor offered reassurance but he ordered a biopsy, just to be certain. She could never have anticipated the outcome of a routine follow-up visit to change the dressings for the biopsy. Her doctor informed Carolyn that she had breast cancer.

"I was all alone at the appointment because I thought I was just there to have the bandages changed. I was so shocked and afraid but I didn't cry. My mom was at my house watching the kids, so I stayed strong. It wasn't until that night that I broke down. My husband and I both cried in the privacy of our bedroom, where the kids wouldn't hear."

Carolyn had a radical mastectomy on November 10, 1965. A few days later, the pathology report indicated that she had cancer in every one of her lymph nodes. The news was devastating for everyone, but Carolyn remained stoic.

"There was some fear but my only thoughts were about my children. They were eighteen months, three, six, nine, and ten years old. My husband was great but he couldn't raise our kids by himself so I knew that I had to live. I knew that I had to stay positive for myself, the children, and my husband. I knew that I couldn't feel sorry for myself."

Once she recovered from surgery, her doctor ordered cobalt treatments five days per week for six weeks. Cobalt is similar to radiation but had a reputation of causing more intense damage to surrounding tissue. It was the only form of treatment available five decades ago and was only offered in a large hospital a fair distance from Carolyn's home. New to the area, Carolyn didn't have a large network of local friends which left only one option for transportation to the hospital.

"My husband was self-employed and we only had one car, so he took off work to drive me to my daily cobalt treatments. We took the three younger kids with us since they weren't in school. He would drop me off at the hospital and take the kids to the park to feed the ducks while I got my treatment."

Each treatment involved lying on a hard wooden table covered with a thin sheet while the cobalt machine hovered over her chest. It was not painful but time consuming, especially with the drive time.

"It was no different than an X-ray but some days took longer than others. I had heard of people having side effects like nausea but I didn't have any ill effects, other than skin discoloration. The hardest part of the treatment was the financial impact. My husband would have to take off a half day and lost a lot of commission but in the end, it made us stronger. What really matters is that those cobalt treatments saved my life."

After six weeks of daily trips to the hospital, Carolyn's journey was complete. She was open about her diagnosis as she wanted to warn others that breast cancer can occur in younger people. She volunteered with Reach to Recovery. It was through the program that she met Jo McCall, a fellow long-term breast survivor in this book.

Carolyn quickly went back to her life as a busy mom, watching her children grow and mature with each passing year.

"Back then, we thought five years was the magic number to be in remission but my breast surgeon never told me I was cured. I saw him twice per year for five years then started going once per year for a mammogram."

She was not given the option of reconstruction so she was fitted with an expensive prosthesis.

"I was happy with the prosthesis and wore one for twenty years. One day, my daughter saw a doctor on television talking about a new form of reconstruction where they use your stomach muscle and tissue. I went to hear him speak but I was nervous about surgery, as I do not tolerate pain medication. My husband told me that I should do whatever I wanted to do for myself, not for him. I decided to have the procedure and I'm so proud of the results. It was a painful recovery but I show off my reconstruction during my mammograms. It was the right choice for me."

Carolyn was the first person in her family to be diagnosed with breast cancer. Her experience enabled her to offer support to other women in her family who have since faced the same disease.

"Seven women in my family had been diagnosed with breast cancer after me. My aunt lived to be almost one hundred years old and my mom lived to the age of eighty-five. My younger sister has survived at least twenty-five years and several of my nieces have been diagnosed."

Carolyn enjoyed many family vacations throughout the years while her children were growing up. They continued the tradition as they each started their own families.

"I rent condos for all of us in Florida and everyone comes together for a week to vacation. It's a great time every year!"

Carolyn has visited her children and grandchildren throughout the United States and as far away as Spain. She has been photographed with several famous actors, made possible through the connections of her granddaughter and her husband. She is very proud of all of her five children, twelve grandchildren, and ten great-grandchildren with one on the way.

"One of my daughters saved my life at a baby shower when she recognized the signs of a stroke. She popped an aspirin in my mouth and took me to the hospital. My husband and I were not highly educated, but my kids are and so are my grandkids. They live all over the world and they are living amazing lives. I'm so proud of all of them."

The anniversary of her diagnosis has been a day of reflection for Carolyn and her family for the last fifty years.

"I think about my journey through breast cancer on that day every year. My sisters call me to tell me they are thankful that I'm still here. I've watched my five children grow up and now they have their own families. My life has been a good one."

Looking back, Carolyn shares her insight as to why she has survived breast cancer for five decades and counting.

"I had a positive attitude and wanted to be there for my five kids. My husband was never a sweet talker but he was very supportive of me. My faith helped me through it and I'm so grateful to my doctor for making the right treatment decisions. The most important thing is to stay positive, I suppose."

Looking to the future, Carolyn plans to continue to enjoy her amazing family. Recently celebrating sixty years of marriage to her husband brought great joy to the entire family. She was pleased to fulfill one last wish this past Christmas.

"I wanted everyone in the family to have dinner together. There were forty-two of us total, from as far away as Ireland and San Francisco. We had a great time together as a family which is a dream come true."

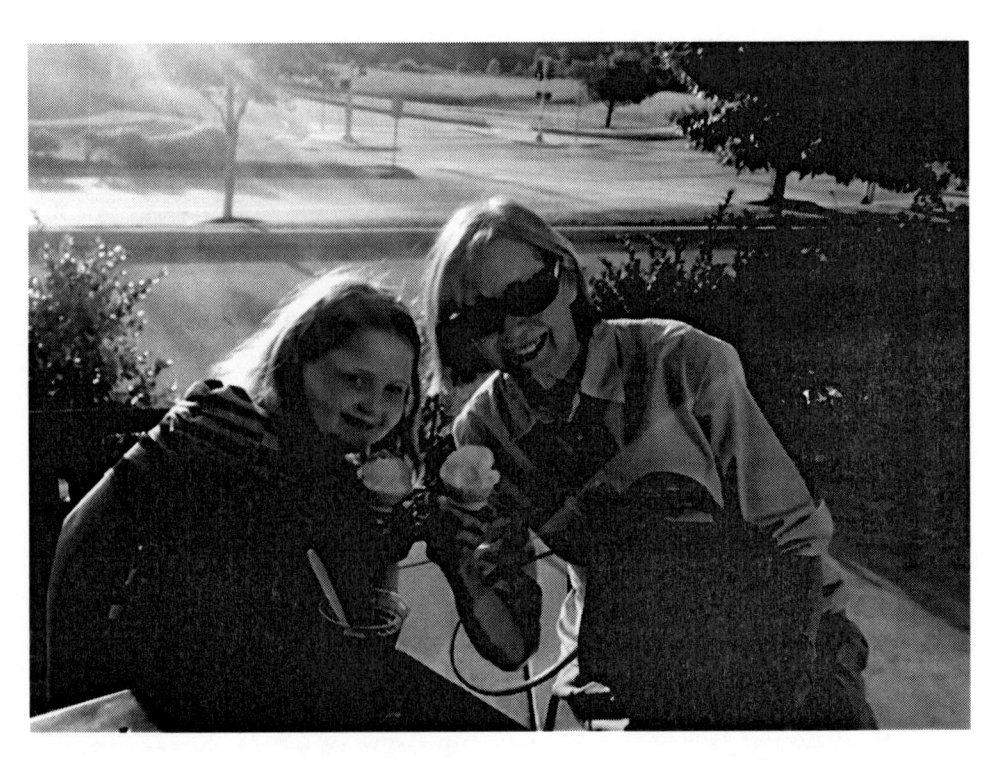

Jo celebrating life with her granddaughter Hanna on their shared birthday!

CHAPTER 13 | Jo McCall

Celebrating Life Since She Was Diagnosed
in November 1974
St. Charles, MO

"I tell women who are facing breast cancer that they have to get in touch with their inner strength. Women are always stronger than they know."

Breast cancer had been a part of Jo's family history for many years. Her paternal grandmother had been diagnosed in 1900 at the age of thirty-one and lost her battle. Her mom was terminally ill due to breast cancer that had metastasized to her lungs. Despite the family history, Jo was healthy and loving life. She was very active at the age of thirty-one, raising two young children, ages two and five.

A novice jogger, Jo noticed a pain in her breast after a run. A quick self-exam revealed a lump which prompted an immediate visit to the doctor.

"The doctor wanted to take a wait-and-see approach. He assured me that the lump would probably go away. I waited six weeks and the lump was still there. I insisted upon surgery to remove it."

Jo was nervous the day of her procedure. She kissed her husband goodbye as the nurses wheeled her into the operating room. Halfway through surgery, the surgeon approached Jo's husband with difficult news. She had breast cancer and they wanted to do a radical mastectomy.

"My husband was faced with a difficult decision. He told them to do the radical mastectomy because he felt that my life was more important than my appearance, especially knowing my family history. It was harder on him than it was me, because he carried the weight of that decision, but it helped knowing that I was completely supportive of his choice."

As Jo slowly came out of anesthesia, her husband told her that she had breast cancer and that he had given the doctor permission to move forward with a mastectomy. Jo was devastated to learn that she had been diagnosed with the same disease that had haunted her life since childhood.

"I cried the entire day after surgery. My kids were so little and I was so afraid. Everyone tried to comfort me, my husband, my roommate in the hospital bed next to me, my nurses. It wasn't until a Reach to Recovery volunteer came to see me that I stopped crying. She was my age with young children and she was a breast cancer survivor. Her visit was very healing for me. I never forgot that woman."

After coping with news of her diagnosis, Jo finally received good news. The tumor was small and had not spread beyond her breast, so surgery was her only form of treatment. While reconstruction was not an option at the time, Jo's scars didn't bother her. She bought a great prosthesis and focused on recovering so she could return to her role as mom to her children.

"I was hopeful but apprehensive about surviving. I didn't have a lot of time to dwell on myself. My mom was losing her battle to breast cancer and needed my help. I focused my time on my mom and my children."

Ten months later, Jo was terrified when she discovered a lump in the scar line of her radical mastectomy. It seemed unfathomable that the breast cancer could have returned so quickly, but tests confirmed the worst. She was diagnosed with a recurrence with six weeks of radiation as the only option for treatment. Maintaining a positive attitude, Jo went back to life as usual.

Remembering the difference the Reach to Recovery volunteer had made for her, Jo waited the mandatory one year after surgery before enrolling in the program. She began visiting women in the hospital after surgery for breast cancer over the next ten years, volunteering as a hospital coordinator for the program that had offered her hope.

"It was so healing to give back to other women. I had never forgotten how much the volunteer helped me after my surgery. I couldn't believe my eyes when she walked into my office building nine years later. I was finally able to thank her for offering the hope that I needed."

She was still volunteering with Reach to Recovery when breast cancer entered her life again, just eight years later. This time, she had a modified radical mastectomy on the other side. She stayed strong through all of it.

"I have a strong inner religious strength. I'm not a big church person, but I lean on God. I love the bible verse, 'When I'm afraid, I put my trust in Thee.' That verse has given me a lot of strength throughout the years."

Surviving breast cancer three times helped bring Jo's marriage closer. It also changed her outlook about what really matters in life. Throughout the years, she has shared specific advice with others, including her sister who was also diagnosed.

"I tell women who are facing breast cancer that they have to get in touch with their inner strength. Women are always stronger than they know. I also tell them to stay busy and positive."

Jo needed to muster all of her strength nineteen years after her second mastectomy. She went in for a routine female exam and discovered that she had Stage

III ovarian cancer. Through genetic testing, she discovered that she has a mutation in her BRCA1 gene. She had chemotherapy and has been cancer free for nearly twelve years.

Jo was first diagnosed with breast cancer more than forty years ago. She has survived breast cancer three times as well as ovarian cancer. Looking back on more than four decades since her diagnosis she shares her thoughts as to why she has lived such a wonderful life since that fateful day in 1974.

"I'm surprised that I am still here, especially after being diagnosed with cancer four times. I didn't do it alone. I had a great medical team and lot of support from friends and family. I've always been brave and positive which is important. I'm very grateful to have a cooperative body with a great healing system."

Jo spent many years with her loving husband who was by her side during her many journeys through cancer. She was there to support him when he was diagnosed with lung cancer five years ago. The cancer metastasized to his brain and he fought for four long brave years. His passing was difficult for the entire family. Jo has slowly adjusted and keeps busy at the young age of seventy-one.

Her children are all grown up now but they live close. Her favorite role in life is grandma to four grandchildren, two boys and two girls.

"There were times when I was concerned that I wouldn't get to meet my grandkids. I am so thankful to be a part of their lives."

Looking to the future, Jo plans to continue spoiling her grandchildren and is considering a riverboat cruise to New Orleans.

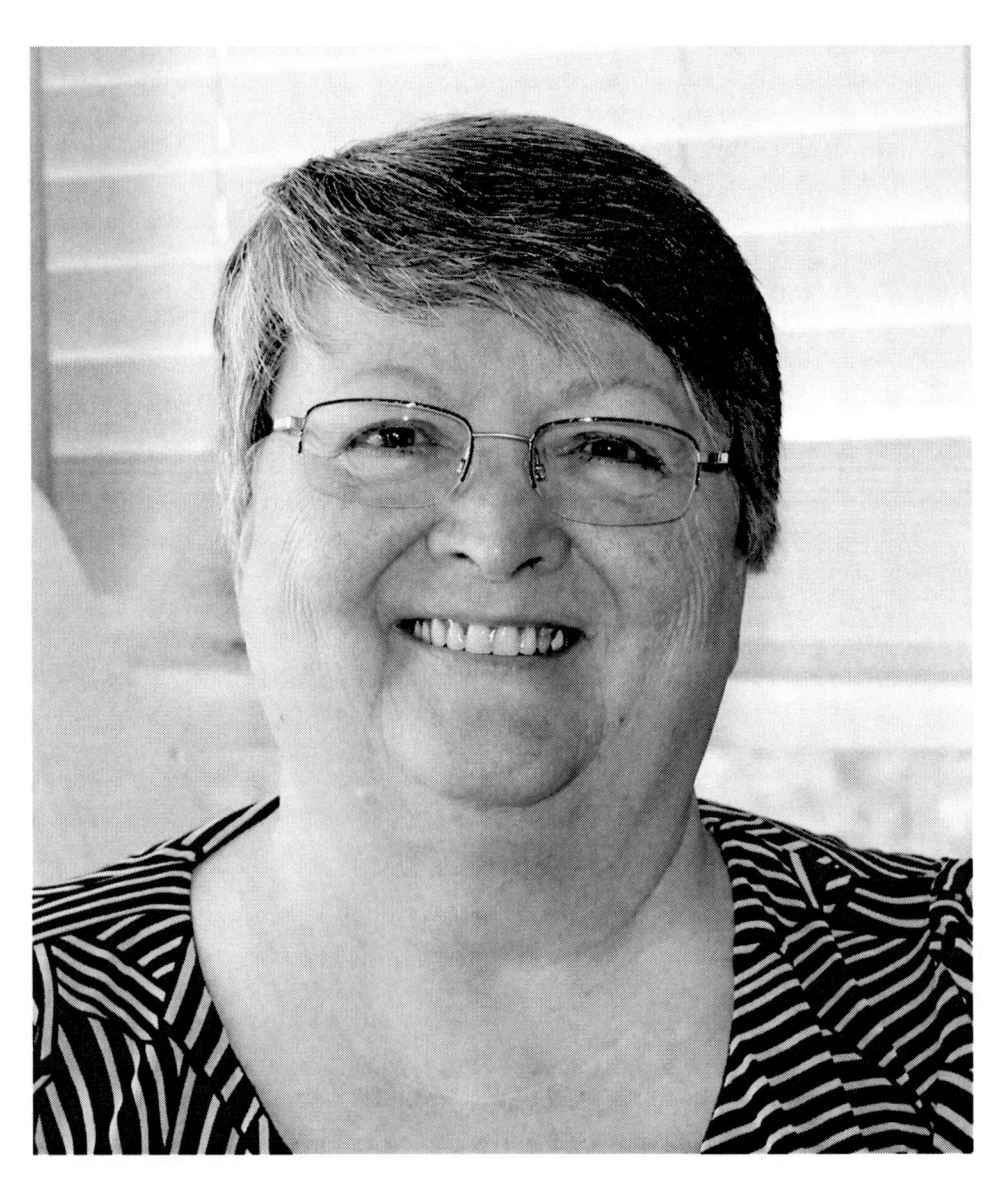

Mary Ellen celebrating life nearly fifty years after breast cancer!

CHAPTER 14 | Mary Ellen Koch

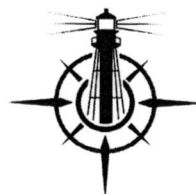

Celebrating Life Since She Was Diagnosed
in January 1966
St. Louis, MO

"Accept what you have to do, then put one foot in front of another and keep on going."

Forced to grow up too quickly, Mary Ellen was orphaned by the age of six years old. Her grandparents and aunt accepted the responsibility of raising both Mary Ellen and her brother, but life was not always easy. She decided to start a new life for herself at the age of twenty-eight.

"I moved across the country to California by myself. I found a job and made a friend which was very exciting. Then, I found a lump in my breast. I was so young but my mother had died from kidney cancer. I knew I needed to see a doctor."

Mary Ellen's doctor sent her for a mammogram which was a much different experience nearly fifty years ago.

"I was taken into a very dark room and a deep voice came out of nowhere, telling me to put 'them' on the table. It was not a good experience for me but we got the films. I waited outside for almost an hour but no one ever came to talk to me so I went home. Things are so different now."

Mary Ellen went back to see her surgeon a few days later. He informed her that she needed to come back after the holidays for a biopsy.

"I had never heard the word biopsy before. My doctor told me the lump was probably nothing because I was too young for breast cancer."

Much has changed in the world of breast cancer detection and treatment, including the biopsy procedure. In Mary Ellen's case, the doctors did a biopsy and examined the frozen section under a microscope. They detected breast cancer cells, so they performed a radical mastectomy immediately. The operation lasted eight hours. Mary Ellen woke up in her hospital room alone.

"When I opened my eyes, I was bandaged from the waist up. I thought it was extreme but what did I know? Then I noticed both of my arms were in a sort of half casts, sticking straight out with my palms facing up. I thought they had dropped me off of the operating table and broken both of my arms."

Following the procedure, the nurses could not answer any of Mary Ellen's questions. She had to wait until that evening for the doctor to confirm her worst fears. He informed her that she had breast cancer and that he had removed her breast and all her lymph nodes.

"I screamed at him! I asked, 'Why did you do this to me?' He looked right at me and told me he did it to save my life."

The doctor wanted Mary Ellen to stay inpatient for two weeks to heal fully from the radical mastectomy. But she had other ideas. With the thoughts of hospital bills looming in her future, she wanted to get back to work. She left the hospital after only one week of recovery.

"When I got home, there was already a hospital bill waiting for me in the mailbox. That was one of the two times that I ever cried about breast cancer. The other time came soon after. I couldn't lift my arms so dressing was difficult. One day, I found myself trapped in my own clothing, half in and half out, unable to move. Luckily a friend arrived to rescue me."

One of the nurses at the hospital told Mary Ellen to use men's t-shirts to absorb the drainage.

"I remember thinking it was bad enough to lose a breast and now they wanted me to wear a man's shirt. I asked a friend's brother to buy some for me. This guy was a prankster. He arrived with a bright red t-shirt with Beethoven's picture on it. He always made me laugh and he was overly supportive. He left a box of doughnuts on my doorstep every other morning."

Mary Ellen continued to heal physically and emotionally.

"I look back now and wonder how I did it. By then, I had gone back to work and was so focused on being able to pay my bills. Once I was done with surgery, I believed it was all over and done with. I didn't have any fear about recurrence because of the lack of information at the time."

Mary Ellen had returned to her job at the bank. She was determined to prove that she could still do her job but she had several unexpected challenges. Her young age in relation to a breast cancer diagnosis raised red flags at the insurance company so they sent someone to observe her at work. Convincing them she was truly recovering from a mastectomy was not difficult as she was still struggling with physical limitations. More apparent was an odd side effect from temporary nerve damage.

"My left arm was still pretty immobile except for when the spasms would hit. It was like an electric impulse shooting through my arm, causing it to fly in the air unexpectedly and do a little dance. At the same time, the pain would cause me to double over and drop whatever was in my other hand. I never knew when the spasms were going to hit and it looked scary. I actually had people run away from me."

The world of prosthetics has changed drastically in the last fifty years. Today, women have many options and entire stores dedicated to mastectomy supplies. But these options were not available for Mary Ellen. She had a hard time finding a store that carried any type of prosthesis.

"Someone referred me to a certain department store and I found a very strange item on display. It looked like a flat bra with two fried eggs for the cups. I was only twenty-eight so I had to work up my courage to ask to see it outside of the case. The elderly clerk called me a pervert which was so humiliating that I left the store."

As prostheses improved throughout the years, they each came with their own unique challenges.

"Years after my mastectomy, I bought a prosthesis that was inflatable. It came with a little straw like the one that comes with a kid's juice box today. It worked well until the day that I got on an airplane. During the flight, the prosthesis started inflating, getting bigger and bigger. I guess it was the air pressure in the cabin. I dashed to the bathroom to deflate myself before I blew up. I can laugh now but it was so embarrassing."

Mary Ellen reflects back on how differently breast cancer was treated nearly fifty years ago.

"Sadly, people were unaware and didn't understand the disease. No one uttered the word cancer. People wouldn't shake my hand because they were afraid of catching it. It was hard because I worked with the public."

Mary Ellen witnessed a dramatic change in breast cancer awareness due to two public figures who shared their story with the world.

"We owe a big thanks to Shirley Temple and Happy Rockefeller for going public with their breast cancer stories. They generated favorable publicity for breast cancer awareness in the early 1970s. They saved a lot of lives with the surge of women who went to the doctor for screenings."

Mary Ellen reached her five-year anniversary of her diagnosis just before Shirley Temple shared her story. She was so happy to reach what was once considered the "magic number" to be cured of breast cancer. She has never experienced a recurrence, but did have a new diagnosis of breast cancer in her other breast forty-seven years after her initial diagnosis.

"This time around has not been a tragedy, but only a bump in the road for me. I had a lumpectomy and thirty-three radiation treatments. The advancements in treatment have made things easier for me. The only thing that really bothers me is that we do not have a real breakthrough or a cure."

Mary Ellen has done her part to help find a cure by participating in two different research studies throughout the years. She has been asked to share her story with others at her cancer clinic and recently gave a speech at a breast cancer event. She conveys her advice for women who have been newly diagnosed.

"Don't overthink it. Accept what you have to do, then put one foot in front of another and keep on going."

She reflects back over her life and offers her insight as to why she has survived breast cancer for nearly fifty years.

"I focused on survival. My prayer throughout both of my illnesses has been, 'Lord help me get through this.' He has . . . twice!"

Looking to the future, Mary Ellen plans to enjoy retirement and spend time with friends and family.

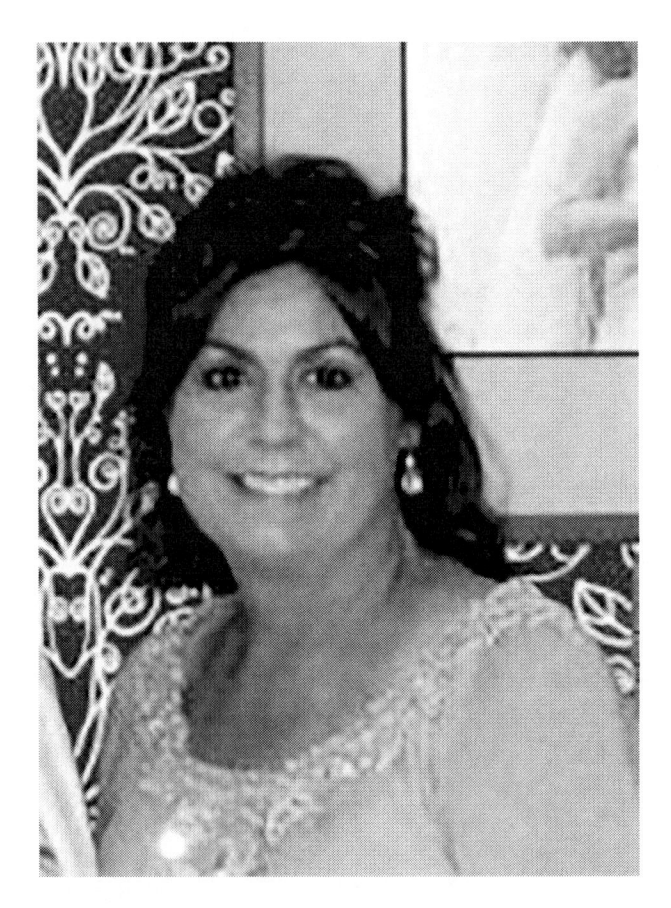

Erin celebrating life nearly twenty-five years after breast cancer!

CHAPTER 15 | Erin Jones

Celebrating Life Since She Was Diagnosed
in May 1991
St. Louis, MO

"I think hope is a big key to be able to look beyond the hard days of treatment. I got through those dark days by focusing on a positive thought for the day. It's easy to feel sorry for yourself, but I knew that I had to be the one to get myself through it."

Erin was living the good life back in 1991. Her hard work and dedication had culminated into a spectacular career with a major insurance company. A full social calendar included many adventures with friends and family. Life was good!

The discovery of a lump under her arm was alarming, but not unfamiliar. Two years prior, Erin had found a similar lump which had been diagnosed as fibrocystic disease after a mammogram and aspiration procedure. She anticipated a repeat performance and wasn't overly worried.

"I didn't have a family history of breast cancer and I was only thirty-three. My doctor tried to aspirate the lump under my arm but instead of fluid this time, there was blood. He told me that wasn't a good sign and ordered an ultrasound."

Erin clung to her belief that it wasn't cancer. Her doctor explained that she needed a surgical biopsy and wanted Erin to sign a consent form giving him permission to do an immediate mastectomy if he discovered cancer during the biopsy. Erin was stunned.

"My mom and sister were with me at the appointment. The doctor told me he thought it was cancer and all I could think was that he didn't know it was cancer. He hadn't even been in there to look at it. I was convinced he was wrong so I decided to get a second opinion before the biopsy. Looking back, I guess I was in denial."

A second opinion resulted in conflicting advice. Erin's second oncologist suggested that she undergo a biopsy, then decide on a treatment plan, even if that meant two separate surgical procedures. Mired in indecision, Erin finally opted to return to her original surgeon. She was in the hospital after surgery when he confirmed her worst fears. Erin had breast cancer.

"I was shocked and more than anything, I was scared. I thought I was going to die. I couldn't believe it. I asked God, 'why me?' It took time but eventually, I had to put it all into perspective."

Still recovering from the biopsy, Erin had a mastectomy one week later. The pathology report brought more difficult news. She had a very aggressive type of breast cancer and it was in at least ten lymph nodes.

"My lymph nodes were all clumped together from the cancer, so it was difficult to determine how many were malignant. That's why I had the lump under my arm. My doctor told me that I had to be aggressive with treatment and suggested chemotherapy and a bone marrow transplant."

Determined to follow her doctor's orders, she drove to a major hospital in Chicago, medical records in hand. The hospital reviewed her case then met with Erin and her family. She was a candidate for a bone marrow transplant and a treatment plan was devised. As fear was replaced with hope, Erin faced an unexpected road block in her journey through breast cancer.

"My insurance company refused to pay for the bone marrow transplant because it was considered experimental. I worked for my insurance company so it was very disappointing. The hospital told me that I could pay for the procedure myself but they wanted the money up front. $230,000!!!! My parents offered to sell their home to pay for it but I couldn't let them do that. We drove back to St. Louis to see my oncologist and came up with a new treatment plan."

A local research-based hospital offered clinical trials which fit with Erin's treatment needs. Following her oncology teams' advice, she opted for an aggressive treatment plan. Conventional chemotherapy would be followed by an experimental trial of high doses of chemotherapy paired with injections to increase her white blood cells. While hopeful for positive results, Erin was faced with a side effect that would alter her future.

"The most difficult part of all of this was just before I started chemotherapy. My doctor told me that I would be sterile after treatment. I had always wanted to have children. It was devastating news but I wanted to live. I told my doctor I was willing to do whatever he recommended to save my life.

Six months of conventional chemotherapy would be challenging for anyone but it was just the beginning for Erin. Enlisting the help of her sister, Erin began the next phase of her treatment regimen.

"My sister would give me shots at home that would increase my white blood cells to more than ten times their normal range. I was admitted to the hospital and started on a three-day chemotherapy drip. It was a very high dose and I received it twenty-four/seven which wiped out my white blood cells, taking them down to almost nothing. I had to wear a mask in the hospital and I was so sick. I spent the entire Christmas holiday and my birthday inpatient, from the Tuesday before Christmas until the day after New Years. My birthday is the day after Christmas so I didn't get to enjoy any part of the holiday that year."

Erin was sent home to recover then started the entire process over again. After injections from her sister at home, she received her chemotherapy drip after being admitted to the hospital. But things didn't go as planned.

"I had one day of the chemo drip when my liver counts went way off. One doctor told me that I probably had breast cancer in my liver. I was terrified. They did a lot of tests and it turns out that my liver was toxic. My body was telling me that it had enough, so in the end, I was two days shy of the full treatment."

Throughout her entire treatment, Erin was determined to live life to the fullest.

"I had planned a road trip with a friend to Chicago to watch the Cardinals play the Cubs. My doctor didn't think it was a good idea but I begged him to let me go. He made me promise to come home if I started running a fever. My friend and I had the best time, going to bars and partying with everyone. I would go to the bathroom and take my temperature to fulfill my doctor's request. I was in the process of losing my hair after my second chemo treatment, so my friend was helping me style it to hide the thin spots. It was such a fun trip even with all of the chaos."

Once chemotherapy was complete, Erin's doctor recommended radiation.

"It seemed like every time I was close to being done with treatment, my doctor would say I needed to do a little more to increase my odds of survival. I did everything he told me to do and focused on a positive outcome. I just kept thinking that it was not going to get me."

Thirty-five radiation treatments completed Erin's treatment.

"I would not be here today if my doctors had not been aggressive. They didn't give up on finding the right treatment which saved my life."

Two years later, Erin had a TRAM flap reconstruction surgery. There is no doubt that the journey through breast cancer changed her life.

"At first, I was worried that people would look at me differently. I never thought I would feel normal again. It took me about ten years to feel like I had beaten it. But I still look at life differently. Even after twenty-four years, I know that I am lucky to be here. I never take things for granted. I live every day like it could be my last and I try to live life to the fullest. I do what makes me happy and focus on the positives in life."

Erin still visits her oncologist for a yearly check up, even though he would have long since discharged her from his care. New pains and blood work cause anxiety but for the most part, breast cancer is now a part of her past.

Reflecting back on her journey, Erin shares her insight as to why she survived breast cancer for twenty-four years and counting.

"My positive outlook is the key. It is part of the healing process. I kept telling myself that I was going to beat this and I believed it. I knew that I wasn't done here on earth. I still had things that I needed to do and I wasn't ready to die. I leaned on my family and friends and my faith throughout the process. I believe that when it's your time to go, you go, but I was determined to fight until the very end."

Times have changed since Erin was first diagnosed. More than two decades ago, people were not as open about breast cancer. It wasn't until her doctor requested that she share her story of survivorship that Erin opened up with other patients.

"I think hope is a big key to be able to look beyond the hard days of treatment. I got through those dark days by focusing on a positive thought for the day. It's easy to feel sorry for yourself, but I knew that I had to be the one to get myself through it."

Looking to the future, Erin plans to continue enjoying time with family and friends. She loves spoiling her nieces and nephews and their children. After planning for years, she enjoyed a trip to New York with her sister. While retirement is far in the future, Erin is looking forward to having more time for travel and volunteer work.

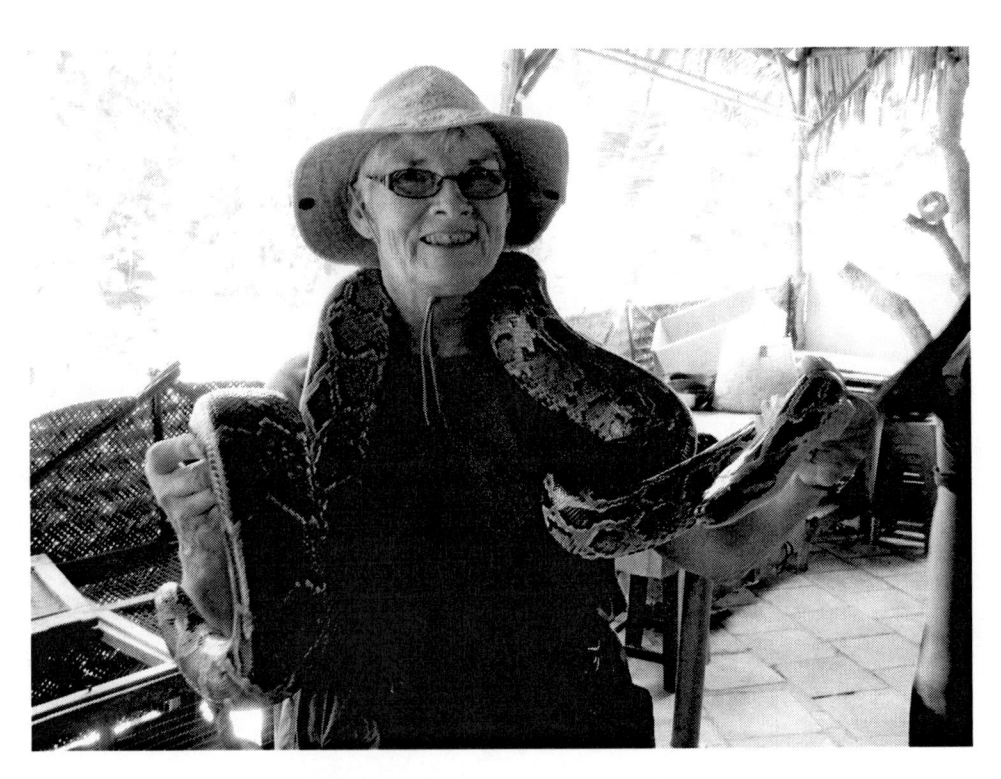

Margaret celebrating life after breast cancer on a trip to Vietnam!

CHAPTER 16 | Margaret Blades

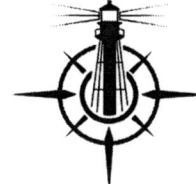

Celebrating Life Since She Was Diagnosed
in February 1974
St. Louis, MO

"I'm sure my kids were terrified when I was first diagnosed, but it made them stronger. It brought all of us closer as a family."

A world traveler at heart, Margaret was enjoying life close to home, raising her young children (ages nine and thirteen) along with her loving husband. Her idyllic life was interrupted one random day when she discovered a lump in her breast. A visit to her obstetrician should have assured her, as he told her it was nothing to worry about. He was confident that she was too young at the age of thirty-three to have cancer and she didn't have a family history.

Margaret shared her doctor's assessment with her husband that evening. They decided to take matters into their own hands and seek a second opinion. Her new doctor sent her to a surgeon. He performed an aspiration procedure in his office. A few days later, Margaret was admitted to the hospital for a biopsy. Concerned about their findings, they immediately performed a modified radical mastectomy and later shared the news that she had breast cancer.

"I think I cried all of the way home. I can still envision that day. My main thoughts were about my children. It was hard to accept. I had done everything right. I had children young, breast fed them, and had no family history of breast cancer. It didn't make sense to me."

Margaret's husband was instrumental in her acceptance of their shocking news. He supported her throughout every step of her journey.

"I knew that breast cancer was a serious diagnosis. I was so afraid that I would never have the opportunity to meet my grandchildren. Times have changed over the last forty years. Back then, very few questions were asked. There was little discussion and patients didn't make many decisions. I think that made it easier in some ways."

Margaret did not have reconstruction and has never wavered on her decision.

"It's not such a big deal to be without a breast. I guess it may depend on your reaction and your husband's reaction but I never felt the need to have reconstruction."

Three weeks after her mastectomy, a severe hail storm offered a distraction for the entire family. It was the first day she had left the house since her surgery.

"The hailstorm was so bad that it broke all the windows in the south side of our home. If I wouldn't have left the house that day, I would have been injured. I was so grateful that I had escaped injury that it shifted my focus. I also had to contend with home repairs after the storm. It was a turning point for all of us."

Margaret's surgery revealed that she did not have lymph node involvement which was a relief to everyone. Her next step was cobalt treatment. Similar to radiation, cobalt had a reputation for being very difficult to tolerate but Margaret handled the treatments without a problem.

"The hardest part of the cobalt treatments for me was relying on others for a ride. My friends and neighbors were quick to volunteer which was nice. I had all of my treatments while my kids were in school so their schedule wasn't affected in any way."

Margaret leaned on her husband, neighbors, and friends throughout her journey, but she never broke the news of her diagnosis to her parents until after the fact.

"Times were different then. I didn't talk to my out-of-town family about breast cancer, especially my dad. He would have thought he had done something wrong if his daughter had breast cancer so we never talked about it."

Once treatment was over, Margaret directed her attention to raising her young children and celebrating life.

"My family had always been big planners, but we started doing things more spontaneously. I'm sure my kids were terrified when I was first diagnosed, but it made them stronger. My husband was so supportive and great with our kids. It brought all of us closer as a family."

Reflecting on her life since her diagnosis, Margaret shares her insight as to why she has survived breast cancer for more than forty years.

"Every time that February thirteenth comes around, we discuss my breast cancer diagnosis and how many years it has been since that day in 1974. I don't really have a formula for having survived for so long. I always stayed busy and tried to enjoy life more every day. It was difficult going through the initial surgery and treatment but you keep meddling along. When you're a mom and have a house to run, you stay busy. That's really my only advice, to stay busy and keep moving forward."

Margaret's family has remained very close. Her son and daughter are adults now and she loves spending time with her three grandchildren. Every year, the entire family goes on vacation together which is always a great adventure.

When not spoiling their grandchildren, Margaret and her husband enjoy traveling throughout the world, which is a true passion for both of them. They have been to all seven continents and 140 countries including Australia and Antarctica.

"My very favorite trip was an African safari. It was fabulous. It was the thing to do! I highly recommend it."

Margaret looks forward to the future with her husband. They plan to continue traveling and spending time with their children and grandchildren for many years to come.

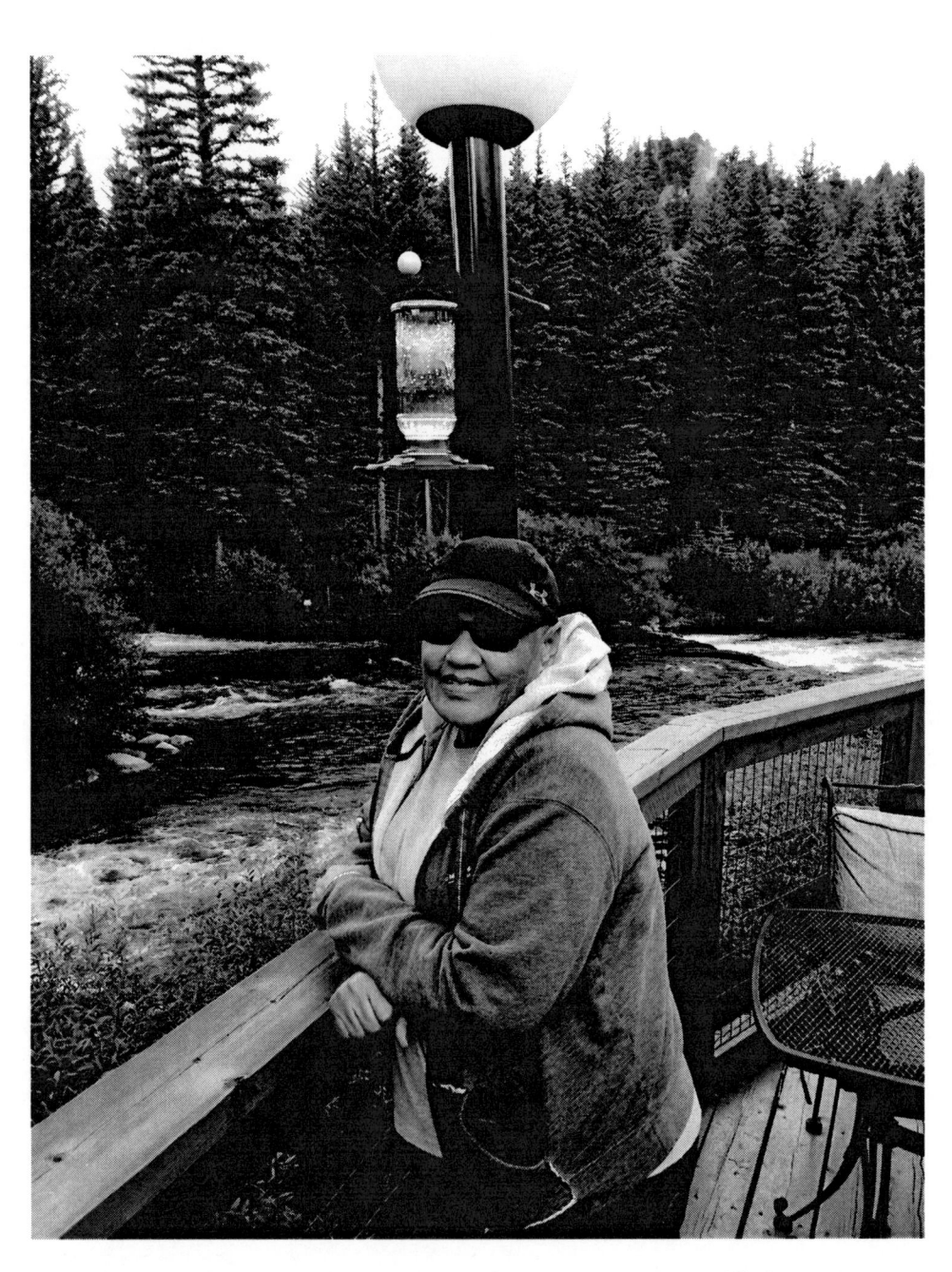

Rhonda celebrating life thirty years after breast cancer on a fun filled vacation!

Chapter 17 | Rhonda Chavis

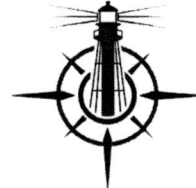

Celebrating Life Since She Was Diagnosed
in June 1985
Harrisburg, Illinois

"I walked three miles the day I was discharged from my mastectomy and went back to work within four weeks of my surgery. I believe that staying active helped me heal."

Exercising and staying active was a lifestyle for Rhonda. She thrived on the adrenaline released from a healthy workout. Walking up to ten miles per day, swimming, running, and biking up to forty miles per day, and lifting weights was the norm. A single mom, she was nearing the end of her daily parenting activities as her youngest was about to graduate from high school.

Breast cancer was no stranger to Rhonda's family. Her aunt had been diagnosed in her thirties but survived until her seventies when she passed away from congestive heart failure. Two cousins had battled metastatic breast cancer. But Rhonda had done everything right. She was selective with her diet, stayed active, and had her children at a young age.

She didn't hesitate to call the doctor when she discovered a large lump in her breast. She waited with bated breath for the biopsy results. Relief washed over her with the news that it was not cancer. But the lump didn't go away. It was painful on occasion, which interfered with Rhonda's love for exercise. Rhonda endured a total of four biopsies, all with the same results before the doctor performed a lumpectomy. Two weeks later, she was summoned to her doctor's office.

"I knew it was cancer when he called me. It turns out there was a spot of cancer hiding behind the big lump. I wasn't given any options other than a mastectomy but my baby was about to graduate from high school. I postponed the surgery for a week so I wouldn't miss graduation."

Rhonda was inpatient for one week after her mastectomy. She was eager to get home and back to work.

"I was walking three miles a day when I was discharged from my mastectomy and went back to work within four weeks of my surgery. I believe that staying active helped me heal. My aunt came to stay with me for that month after surgery to help cook and clean which was amazing. The hardest part was wearing the prosthesis so soon, but I managed."

Rhonda's family and friends offered love and support throughout her journey. She never doubted that she would survive after watching her aunt live a long, happy life for decades after diagnosis. She leaned heavily on her faith and prayed for strength to get through the difficult days.

"I never let breast cancer stop me from doing anything I wanted to do. I went back to riding my bike, lifting weights, and running."

Rhonda's passion for staying active and her insight into the importance of the health benefits of exercise led her start a revolution at work.

"I started a movement at work that encourages people to walk on their lunch break. Staying active is vital to everyone's health. I tell people to take one day at a time and stay positive."

Once she moved past the initial fears of recurrence, Rhonda went on with life. As her role of motherhood changed with her children leaving home, she started thinking about finding new love. But she was concerned about her appearance. Her body image suffered as a result. Until a wonderful man walked into her life. They fell in love and married eleven years after her diagnosis. They are still happily married today.

Rhonda's struggle with her body image led to the decision to have reconstructive surgery twenty years after her mastectomy. Her new body image gave her the confidence to accomplish a long-desired goal in life.

"I was always self-conscious about what tops I wore because of the prosthesis. After twenty years of not having a breast, I had reconstruction. That gave me the courage to learn to swim. I had always wanted to learn but I waited until my late fifties to do it. That's when I decided to do a sprint triathlon."

Rhonda and her husband were looking forward to an active life after retirement when she was diagnosed with colorectal cancer in 2010. The doctors informed her that this cancer was not related to her original breast cancer diagnosis. The treatment process including surgery, chemotherapy, and radiation, have been challenging but she continues to have a positive attitude.

"I have pain from the colorectal surgery but we are working to relieve that pain with a neuro-stimulator. My husband and I recently enjoyed a vacation in Colorado and had a great time."

Reflecting back on her life since her breast cancer diagnosis, Rhonda shares her insight as to why she has survived breast cancer for three decades and counting.

"My aunt was a great role model for long-term survival which helped me stay positive. I truly believe this is the key to surviving cancer and living a long life. Staying positive is so important. I also leaned on my faith, support from family and friends, and had a great medical team. My active, healthy lifestyle helped me recover from treatment."

Today, Rhonda enjoys spending time with her grown children and stepchildren as well as her grandchildren. Her husband continues to shower her with love and support.

Looking to the future, Rhonda hopes to accomplish one more major physical challenge with her husband.

"I want to bike ride across the country. Years ago, I biked across the state of Indiana which spurred the idea to bike across the entire country. I have to heal and get past the pain from surgery first, but cancer has never stopped me from doing anything before and it won't stop me now."

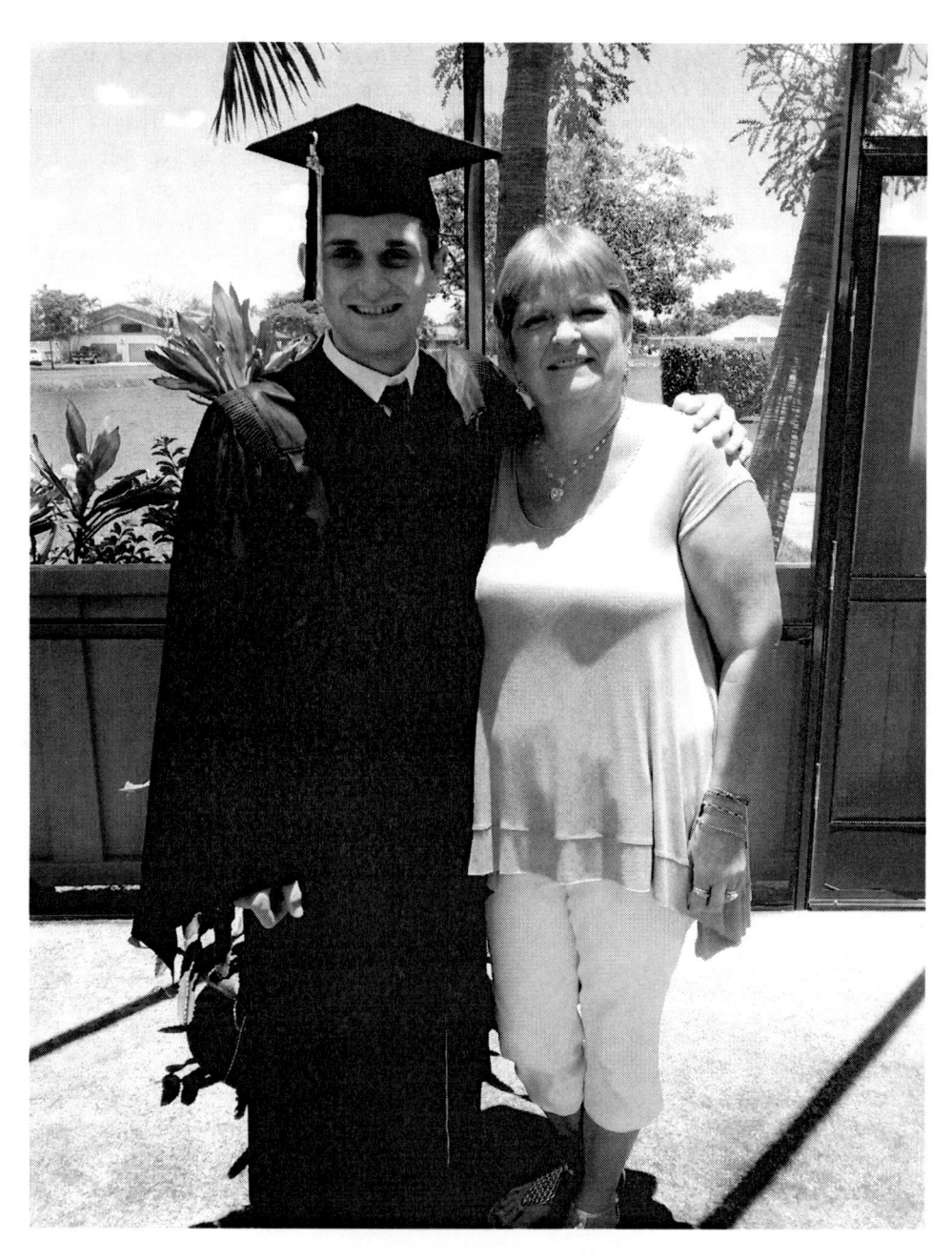

Cheryl celebrating life after breast cancer with her oldest grandson, Gage, at his high school graduation!

CHAPTER 18 | Cheryl Coomes

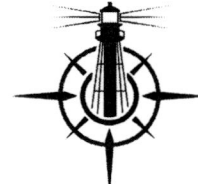

Celebrating Life Since She Was Diagnosed
in September 1990
Boca Raton, FL

"Breast cancer changed my life for the better. I realized how precious life is and how quickly it can be taken from you. I appreciate waking up every morning and live life to the fullest."

Life was busy for Cheryl as a wife and mom to four children, ages eight, twelve, and sixteen and a stepson who was thirteen. In addition to the hustle and bustle of parenthood, Cheryl was struggling with the side effects of a hysterectomy at a young age. Determined to help alleviate her symptoms, her doctor prescribed hormone replacement medication, quadrupling the dose within the first month. One month later, a large lump appeared in Cheryl's breast.

"I showed it to a close friend at work and she was scared. I left work and went to the doctor that day. I didn't return to work for a year. It was all such a whirlwind."

Cheryl had dense breast tissue and a history of fibrocystic lumps. This new lump was never detected by a mammogram but the ultrasound confirmed that something was amiss. Her doctor contacted a surgeon with a request for immediate surgery.

"There was disagreement between my doctor and the surgeon. My doctor insisted that I needed surgery, but the surgeon said I was too young to have breast cancer and I didn't have a family history."

The surgeon relented and performed the biopsy.

"I was in the hospital after surgery when my surgeon walked in. He couldn't look me in the eye as he told me that I had breast cancer. It was a desperate, hopeless feeling. I began to cry and scream so they moved me into my own room. I thought it was a death sentence and I had children at home."

Diagnosed with Stage III breast cancer that was moving into Stage IV, the only option was a radical mastectomy and a complete lymph node dissection. It was a difficult surgery but time was of the essence. Her incision were still healing when Cheryl began a rigorous course of chemotherapy.

"I would stay in the hospital for three weeks at a time for each chemo treatment. I would go home for a week and then head back to the hospital for the next treatment. This went on for an entire year. The worst part was that I had to be quarantined from my children. My youngest was eight years old, so she went to live with her grandma. The side effects were rough but missing my kids was the worst part. I remember lying in the hospital, staring out the window, day after day. I was afraid that I would never get to meet my grandchildren."

Cheryl's husband was loving and supportive throughout her entire treatment. He enjoyed her sense of humor during the hardest days, including the way she coped with losing her long, beautiful hair.

"I knew my hair was going to fall out, so I dyed it purple. My husband just laughed. As soon as it started falling out, I took control by having my hairdresser shave it. I lost every bit of my hair but he never cared."

Cheryl's sister lived far away but she was determined to offer much-needed support.

"My sister, Linda, would fly in from out of state to be with me. She was an instrumental part of my healing."

Once the difficult year of chemotherapy was completed, Cheryl started radiation. Concerned about the high possibility of recurrence, her doctor's recommended a prophylactic radical mastectomy on the other side. Cheryl was determined to do everything possible to survive so she complied with her doctor's recommendation.

"I never had reconstruction and I miss shopping for bras at Victoria's Secret. But I have a great prosthesis and I can look past the scars."

After healing from her second radical mastectomy, it was time to move past breast cancer. Like so many women, Cheryl struggled with this transition.

"I was freaked out at first. I wanted the doctor to watch over me. But that fear lessened with time and I learned to appreciate every day."

With a new understanding of the true impact of a cancer diagnosis, Cheryl wanted to give back to others. She volunteered for Reach to Recovery, enjoying visiting and inspiring women after surgery for breast cancer. She also shares support and gifts with neighbors and friends who have been touched by cancer.

"I tell others who are facing breast cancer that it's okay to cry but always focus on the positive."

Strengthened by her journey, Cheryl faced another, more frightening health scare nine years after her breast cancer diagnosis. A brain aneurism brought her to the brink of death, but she made a full recovery. Cheryl is confident this is a second reason to believe that God has a plan for her.

"I made it through breast cancer and an aneurysm. Breast cancer made me appreciate my life, but the brain aneurysm canceled any lingering doubts about having a reason to be on this earth. I woke up in the hospital and the doctor told me, 'Yes ma'am, you should be dead.' Two weeks later, I was back at the office working."

Today, Cheryl stays active with her family and continues to lavish her sense of humor on those closest to her. Her children have been on their own for many years and have blessed her life with eight grandchildren, one of whom lives with her. Her heart is filled with gratitude every time she spends time with the grandchildren she wasn't sure she would ever meet.

"Breast cancer changed my life for the better. I realized how precious life is and how quickly it can be taken from you. I look in the mirror and see scars, but I can look past them. I appreciate waking up every morning and live life to the fullest."

She commemorated her twenty-year survivor celebration at a big event in Fort Lauderdale. She signed the pink fire truck and wore a pink shirt that said "Twenty-Year Survivor." However, there are many years that her anniversary dates goes by without acknowledgment.

Looking back, Cheryl shares her insight as to why she believes she has survived breast cancer for more than two decades.

"My positive attitude and sense of humor helped me survive. My faith and prayers were also important. A few years ago, my fifteen-year-old grandson looked me in the eye and said, 'All of those years ago, God knew that I would need you.' He is right . . . God had a reason for me to be here."

Cheryl's bucket list includes a visit to New York to see the Statue of Liberty and Central Park. She plans to retire, continue to travel and spoil her grandchildren. She looks forward to becoming a great-grandmother someday in the future.

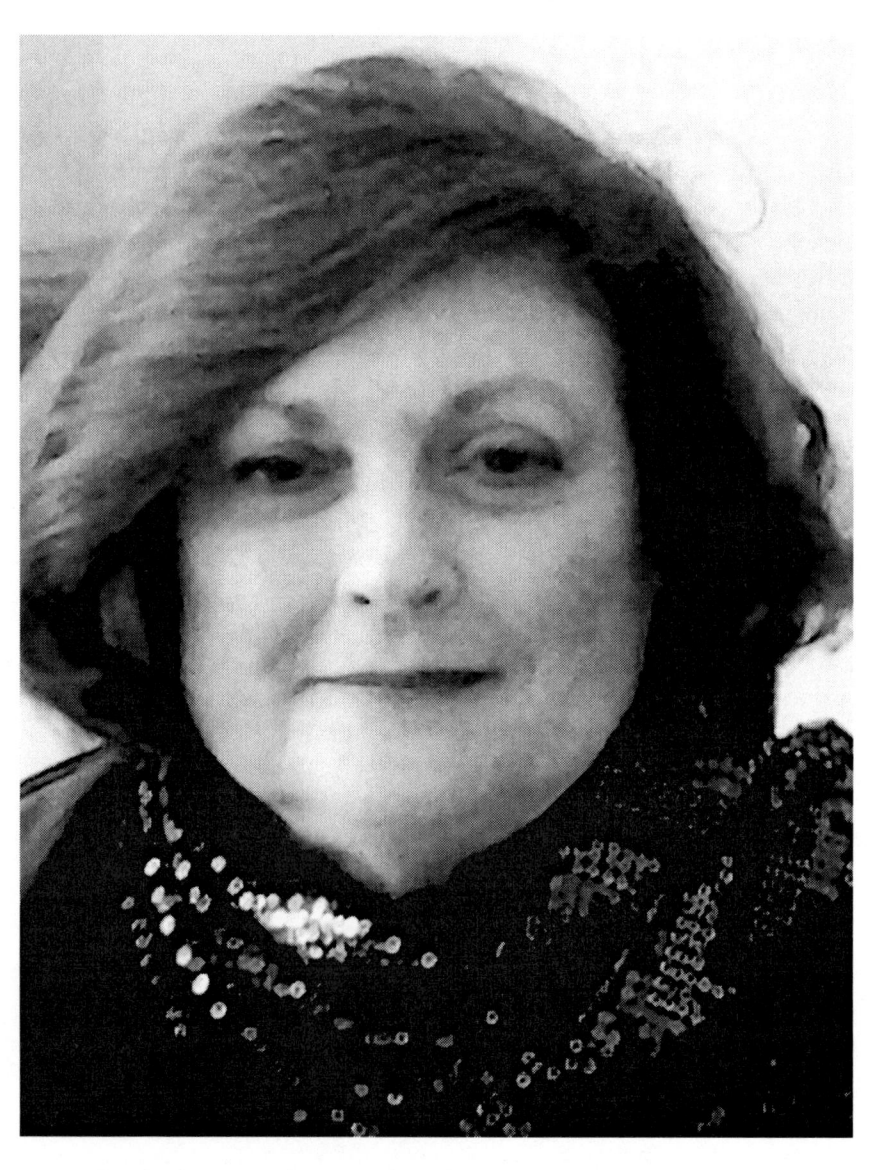

Rosalind enjoying life more than three decades after breast cancer!

CHAPTER 19 | Rosalind Steel

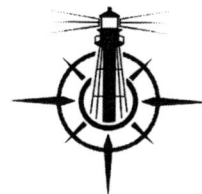

Celebrating Life Since She Was Diagnosed
in November 1982 and 2010
St. Louis, MO

"I was wearing bunny slippers, dancing in the hospital as I was scrubbing my body for surgery."

New beginnings seemed to be a guiding force in Rosalind's life back in 1982. In the midst of working on her Master's degree, she was focused on taking her teaching career to the next level. Busy was an understatement, as she was working full time and still recovering from a divorce from three years prior. In spite of everything, Rosalind was finding happiness in the world on her own.

One day, while lying on her stomach, Rosalind discovered a small, hard lump in her breast. It was new, no doubt, as she had been to the gynecologist for a clinical exam the month before.

Putting one of her teaching tools to good use, she circled the lump with a black magic marker and went to see her gynecologist the next day.

"I went to see a surgeon who did a biopsy in his office. He didn't tell me at the time, but he knew it was breast cancer. He waited until the pathology report confirmed his belief. I had breast cancer."

Rosalind's surgeon recommended a mastectomy but Rosalind wanted a second opinion.

"I went to see another doctor for a second opinion and he yelled at me. 'Do you want to lose your breast or die?' I wasn't upset about losing my breast, I only wanted a second opinion. In the meantime, my original doctor was upset that I got a second opinion. He tried to schedule the surgery without my consent. I was so upset that I walked out of his office and never returned. I was a recently divorced woman living alone and had left the only doctor that I'd ever known. I didn't tell anyone in my family and tried to figure it all out on my own."

Rosalind was reeling with the news of her diagnosis and finally confided in her two best friends.

"I told them that I didn't want any crying or moping. I needed their help to find a new doctor. Fate was on my side, as my friend shared my story with a customer and he referred me to a great breast specialist. I knew that he was the right doctor for me as soon as I met him."

Rosalind's new surgeon insisted that she needed support, despite her concern about burdening her friends and family with her upcoming surgery. She relinquished and shared her news. Everyone was supportive including her professors who allowed her to postpone her last exam for her Master's degree until after surgery.

"I had so much support. Friends and family decorated my room the night before surgery and we partied together. I was wearing bunny slippers, dancing in the hospital as I was scrubbing my body for surgery."

The partial mastectomy procedure led to the discovery of cancer in her lymph nodes and a lymph node dissection. Recovering at her parents' home gave Rosalind time to contemplate her treatment plan which included two weeks of radiation followed by two years of chemotherapy.

"They injected the chemotherapy into the back of my hand. It was spooky to watch it entering my body very slowly. It didn't hurt but the smell would make me queasy. I was so calm on the exterior and reassured my fellow patients who were getting chemotherapy. The nurses often mistook me for the friend of a patient because of my attitude."

Determined not to bother her family and friends, Rosalind went to most of her chemotherapy appointments alone. Daily treatments after work for one week were followed by three weeks off, then the cycle would repeat over the course of two years.

"My friends and family were a great support system but I wanted them to know that I was okay and didn't need their help with the chemotherapy. I felt strong enough to handle it on my own."

Life went on during those two years of treatment. Rosalind graduated with her Master's degree and she adjusted to new medical professionals after her radiologist and surgeon moved. Once her chemotherapy regime was complete, she was given a clean bill of health. She worked hard in the education field, changing her students' lives through her career as an assistant principal.

"Other things in life changed my life much more than breast cancer. But one positive that came out of my diagnosis was that I was brought back to my faith. The first time I went to church, tears started rolling down my face. I kept going back for more and later joined the choir. I find great comfort in being closer to God."

In 2010, twenty-eight years after her initial diagnosis, breast cancer made another appearance in Rosalind's life.

"A mammogram detected cancer in the same breast but it was not connected to my first breast cancer. This new cancer had already moved into my skin and was headed toward my other breast."

Rosalind initially had a unilateral mastectomy then one month later went in for a mastectomy on the other side. The surgeries were extensive in order to obtain clean margins. Reconstruction is not an option, due to skin involvement. Rosalind remains positive and upbeat about the results of her multiple surgeries.

"I don't look at my body as deformed. I look at it as having gone through a trauma. I usually drape a scarf across my chest to hide the fact that I don't wear a prosthesis."

Rosalind remained in the field of education throughout her life until she retired fourteen years ago. She has a strong network of friends who can relate to her health struggles over the years. She has also had in-depth conversations with her sister about both of their cancer experiences.

Reflecting upon the more than three decades since her diagnosis, Rosalind shares her insight about why she has survived breast cancer twice and is still going strong.

"It was in the cards. I know that worrying about cancer won't cure it. You have to go on with life. I celebrated the anniversary for the first twenty years after my diagnosis but that was my mental cut-off point. It was time to move on. Life goes on around you and you have to keep on moving."

Rosalind has enjoyed time in London and many special moments with family and friends. Over the years, Rosalind has volunteered with several wild animal rescues fueling her passion for animals. She has enjoyed feeding wolves at the Wolf Sanctuary and most recently had a once-in-a-lifetime experience.

"I got to feed a rescued baby white Bengal tiger. I've had some really great experiences in my life and you never know what's around the corner. I have a lot of fun and I'm full of life. I appreciate the big things and the small ones. What else can I want out of life? I'm happy with the surprises that God had for me."

Looking to the future, Rosalind would love to help someone else who is going through breast cancer. She plans to enjoy many more adventures with her friends and her beloved cat, Jasper.

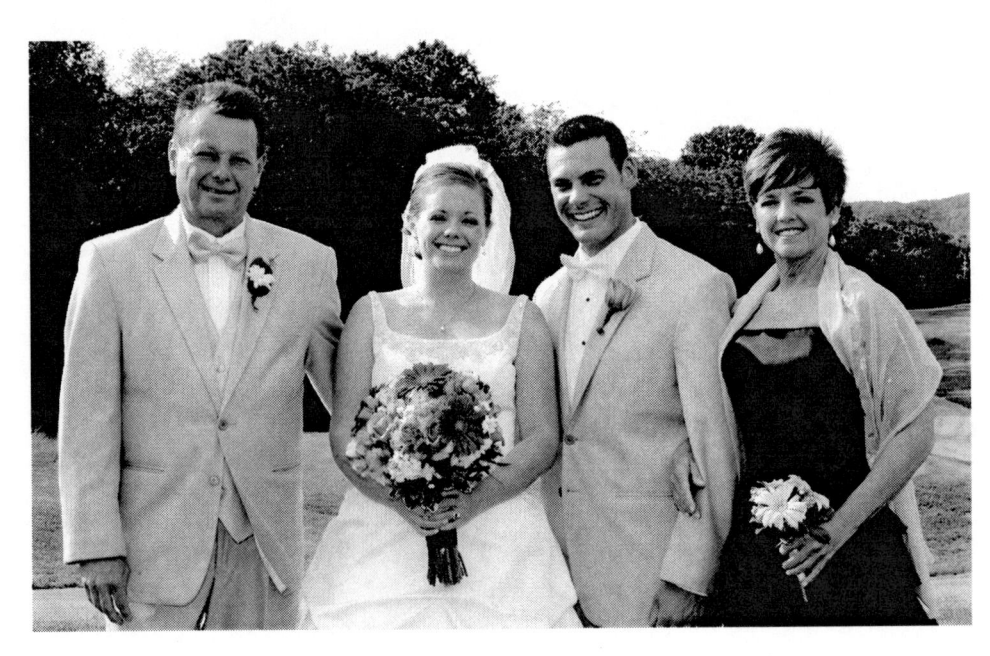

Lisa celebrating life after breast cancer at her daughter, Kelly's wedding!

CHAPTER 20 | Lisa Cushing

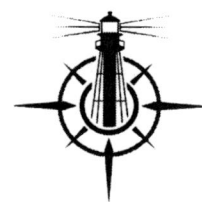

Celebrating Life Since She Was Diagnosed
in January 1985
Eureka, MO

"I would go to treatment then to work. It wasn't easy, but what else was I supposed to do? I wasn't going to lie down and die. I just kept moving forward."

Lisa was loving life with her husband and two-and-a-half-year-old little girl. Like many moms, she was engaged in the delicate balance of motherhood and a full-time career at the age of twenty-six. In the midst of preparing for the Christmas season, she discovered a lump in the upper quadrant of her breast.

"My breasts were always lumpy during my period but the lumps always went away. This one felt different so I called my doctor."

Lisa's doctor advised her to wait two weeks due to her age and history of bumpy breasts around her cycle. After waiting the prescribed time, she saw a surgeon who tried unsuccessfully to drain the lump. A biopsy was performed and everyone waited with bated breath for the results.

"My husband woke to me crying in bed. My doctor had called very early that morning with the results of my biopsy: breast cancer. I was so young and had a little girl. I've always been a positive person and all I could think was let's get this done and take care of it."

Treatment decisions followed the diagnosis. Lisa weighed the option of a lumpectomy or mastectomy, having been assured by her doctor that the survival rates were the same for either option. She opted for a lumpectomy. The pathology report held both good and challenging news. The cancer was contained within the tumor but it had spread to one of thirty lymph nodes. Her surgeon consulted with a specialist before recommending the next phase of treatment: one year of chemotherapy followed by eight weeks of radiation. Lisa maintained her routine throughout treatment.

"My job had the health insurance so it never occurred to me to quit. My husband and daughter needed me so I would go to treatment then to work. It wasn't easy, but what else was I supposed to do? I wasn't going to lie down and die. I just kept moving forward."

Lisa maintained a positive attitude throughout her year of treatment.

"I never lost my hair, so I didn't look like a typical breast cancer patient. My chemo was given in the form of an injection. It burned my veins intensely so the nurses would give it to me slowly. My white blood count would drop immensely so we would have to delay my bimonthly treatments. I also had eight weeks of radiation. My biggest side effect was being tired."

One of Lisa's biggest supporters has been her husband of more than thirty-three years. He has been there for her every step of the way.

"My husband was great through all of it, but he never really saw me that sick. I went to work every day and never lost my hair. If you ask him, he didn't see breast cancer as a huge challenge because of how I handled treatment."

Toward the end of chemotherapy, Lisa's in-laws treated her family to Hawaii for two weeks.

"I loved that vacation. It was so very beautiful and healing for me."

She also fulfilled a dream of building a house with her husband. Facing a breast cancer diagnosis and the treatment that followed was a challenge, but Lisa discovered many positive outcomes as well.

"Breast cancer changed my life by making me stronger. I never take life for granted because life is short. I am more patient and humble than before breast cancer. I try to live life with no regrets."

Lisa has been grateful for many things over the last three decades, but the opportunity to raise her daughter and be a part of her grandchildren's lives has brought her overwhelming joy.

"Watching both of my grandchildren be born is the highlight of my life. I was in the delivery room with my daughter up until the moments before each of her babies were born. It was such an emotional day for me. Both times, I flashed back to the day I was diagnosed when I wanted more than anything to survive breast cancer and watch my baby grow up. That special moment in life when my grandchildren were born was more meaningful to me because I appreciate every day of life more than the average person."

Lisa has often been a source of inspiration for other women facing a breast cancer diagnosis. She shares the following advice with those going through treatment.

"Make sure you find a doctor that you like and trust. Don't settle for someone that you don't trust with your life. It's your body, so do what's right for you. Stay away from negativity and focus on the positive. Do everything you can to help yourself and keep fighting."

Reflecting on the last thirty years of her life, Lisa shares her insights as to why she has survived for three decades and counting.

"I have always been a very positive, upbeat person and make it a point to avoid negativity. I think it helped that I have remained physically active through the years, running, walking, and lifting weights. I take a mental break from life while running and tune into my own thoughts as a form of therapy. I also have a personal relationship with God. I'm so thankful to Him for giving me the strength to battle breast cancer and the many blessings in my life."

Looking to the future, Lisa plans to continue spoiling her grandchildren and enjoy time with her husband.

CHAPTER 21 | Tonya Salkowski

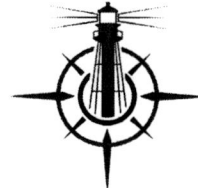

Celebrating Life Since She Was Diagnosed
in August 1994
St. Louis, MO

"It's so important to find a doctor that is positive. I found a new oncologist because my first one made me feel down when I left. I tell women to be strong and do what they need to do to get through it."

Tonya had orchestrated a perfect life for herself. She had found a balance between motherhood to her seven-year-old daughter, spending time with her devoted husband, and a job that she fed her passion: teaching aerobics. Breast health was a part of her busy life with her history of having a benign lump removed in the past and her lumpy, bumpy breasts. She had also witnessed both her mother and grandmother have positive outcomes from breast biopsies. She wasn't overly concerned when her doctor found a lump in her breast during a routine exam.

Although her doctor recommend a follow-up appointment with a surgeon, Tonya decided to take a wait-and-see approach. After a year and a day, she had an overwhelming feeling that she needed to have a mammogram. Following her instinct, she went to see a surgeon. He alleviated any concern with news that her mammogram was fine and was quick to point out that she was too young for breast cancer. All signs pointed to the probability that the lump was fatty tissue, but her surgeon performed a needle biopsy, just to be safe.

Still unconcerned, Tonya was working a few days later when her husband walked into her office unexpectedly. His face reflected his concern as he asked if she had heard the news. Her life changed as her husband shared the doctor's report. Tonya had breast cancer.

"At first, I had no reaction at all. The phone rang so I answered it. I listened as my doctor told me that I had breast cancer. My husband held me as I sat in my cubicle and cried for a few minutes. I dried up my tears and said 'Let's go to lunch.' I never cried again."

Before the shock of diagnosis wore off, Tonya had to make treatment decisions. Her surgeon offered the option of a lumpectomy or mastectomy. This was an easy decision for her.

"I knew too many stories of women who had lumpectomies and the cancer came back. I decided that I wanted to do everything possible to stop the cancer the first time around. I opted for a unilateral mastectomy without reconstruction."

Still recovering from surgery, Tonya was inundated with challenging news from the pathology report. Four of her lymph nodes tested positive for cancer. Her doctor estimated a 95% chance of recurrence. Faced with eight rounds of chemotherapy, Tonya wore a brave face, determined to survive.

"The nausea from chemotherapy was not controlled by the medications prescribed by my doctor. I started seeing a holistic chiropractor who had studied in China. She would alter my diet based on blood work after each chemotherapy treatment. I also had acupuncture treatments which helped with the side effects."

As expected, the chemotherapy caused hair loss, but Tonya took it in stride. Her husband shaved her head when hair began to fall out and she had a great time trying on wigs. She never left home without her wig, reveling in her new hairstyle. As many breast cancer survivors will attest, wearing a wig can bring unexpected adventure at times.

"We were running through the airport, trying to catch a flight to Hawaii for our family vacation. People kept staring at me and I thought it was because I was running. When we got to the gate, my husband looked at me and started laughing. My wig was falling off of my head from running so fast. That story still makes us laugh all of these years later."

Seven weeks of radiation followed chemotherapy which was uneventful in terms of side effects. Although experimental at the time, Tonya's doctor prescribed Tamoxifen. The side effects were challenging over the next two years but when it caused her blood pressure to increase, Tonya's doctor told her to stop taking it. She opted for a hysterectomy based on the knowledge that her cancer was hormone driven.

Tonya leaned on her faith during her journey through breast cancer and throughout her life.

"I believe that God helps those who help themselves. I have to do everything that I can and the rest is in God's hands. I talk to God but I also accept His will. I had a lot of people praying for me and I appreciated that."

Breast cancer changed Tonya's life in many ways. After being physically fit for her entire life, she struggled with the side effects of treatment when exercising. She had to give up teaching aerobics but it was a small price to pay for living the next twenty years cancer free.

"My husband was my rock through all of my treatment. He would take care of everything so that I could focus on getting better. I always knew that he was strong but now I know he will always be there for me. I feel closer to my family and it reinforced my belief that I am a strong person."

Many women struggle after treatment ends, but Tonya decided to look to the future. She was never a believer in statistics, so her doctor's warning that she had a 95% chance of recurrence fell on deaf ears. Tonya followed up with her oncologist for five years and hasn't seen one since then.

As she reflects back on the last twenty-one years, she shares her insight into why she has survived breast cancer for decades.

"I think that my positive attitude helped me survive as well as taking action. I did everything that I could do to keep it from coming back. I try to keep stress out of my life. Stress impacts the body so much then your defenses are down and the cancer is able to attack."

Tonya often talks to and supports other women who are going through breast cancer. She shares advice and insight based on her own journey.

"It's so important to find a doctor that is positive. I found a new oncologist because my first one made me feel down when I left. I tell women to be strong and do what they need to do to get through it but be open with your doctor. I was really struggling after my first chemotherapy treatment but I was trying to be strong. I went in for my second treatment and he told me that I should always call with symptoms. He gave me medication to help counteract the symptoms and I tolerated the second treatment so much easier."

Today, Tonya works with her husband at their printing and mailing service company. Her daughter is all grown up now and works with her parents at their company. She is happily married and recently gave birth to a perfect baby boy named Landon.

Looking to the future, Tonya hopes to move to Hawaii. Beyond the beauty and the weather, she feels better physically when on the island. She is looking forward to retiring and spoiling her grandson.

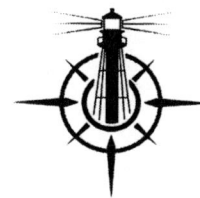

SECTION 3
Faith in God, Self, and Others

Facing our own mortality is life changing. In the times of darkest despair, many of us to turn to faith. The long-term survivors in this section share stories of leaning on faith in God, self, and others to overcome their fears and challenges on their journey through breast cancer and beyond.

A deep spiritual faith in God carried many of the women through their darkest days. Others found comfort in their relationships with spouses and friends. Still others found a way to dig deep into their own psyche to move past breast cancer.

As you immerse yourself in the faith of the women in these chapters, I invite you to explore your own faith in a higher being, self, and others. How has your faith been strengthened or challenged through your journey?

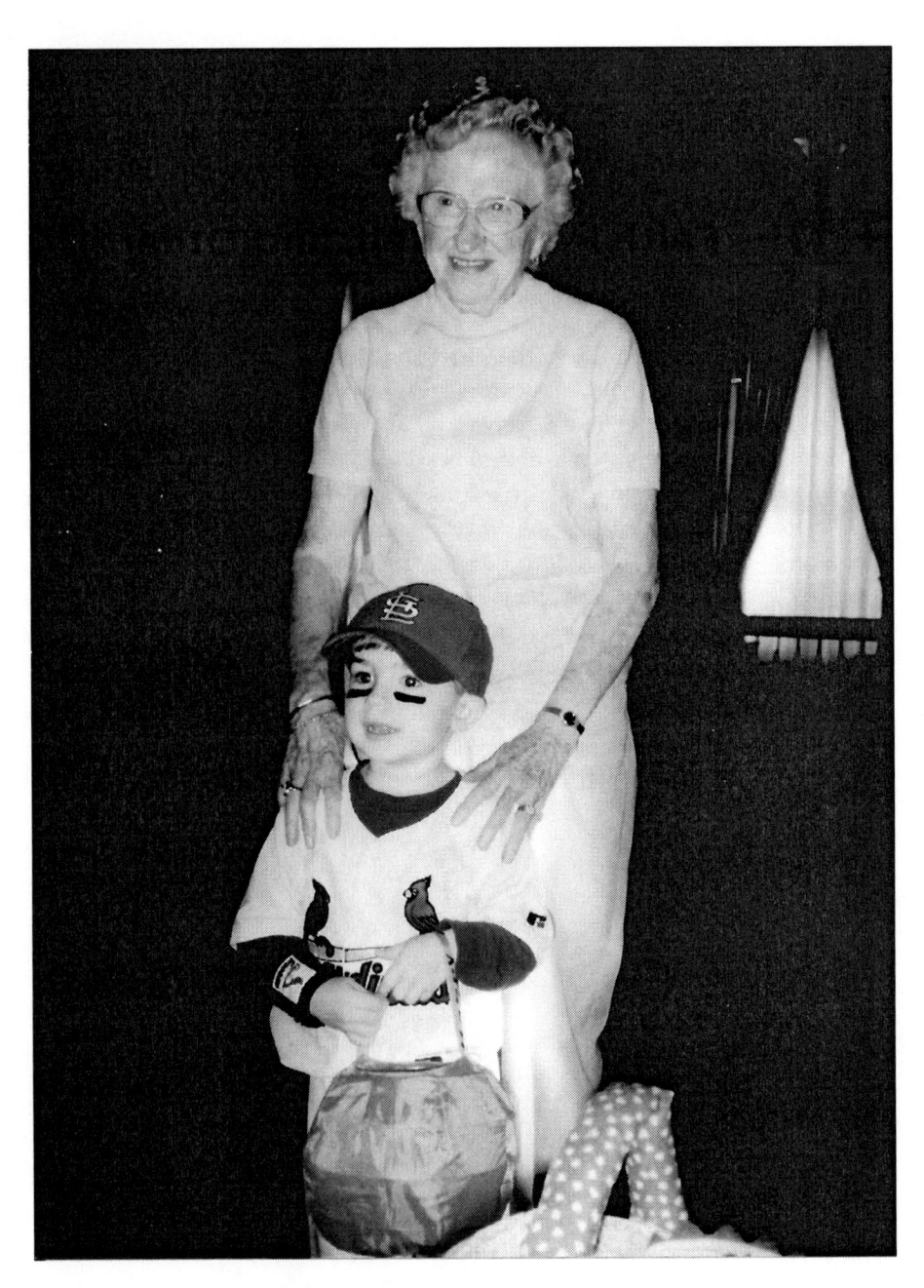

*Grace celebrating life after breast cancer with one of three
great-grandchildren who have blessed her life!*

Chapter 22 | Grace Allen

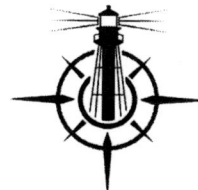

Celebrating Life Since She Was Diagnosed
in 1972
Jerseyville, IL

"I took one day at a time and then I would suddenly realize that I hadn't thought about breast cancer for a day, a week, and then a month. You don't ever forget it but it does get easier."

Life was wonderful for Grace and her husband. Just shy of turning fifty, she was enjoying an exciting phase in life as a new grandparent with another grandbaby on the way. She was excitedly preparing for a trip with her husband when she found a lump in her breast. Somehow, deep down, Grace knew it was breast cancer. She was familiar with the disease as both her mother and grandmother had lost their battle with breast cancer.

"I was terrified but I knew that sharing my news would ruin our trip. I kept the lump a secret for the next four days. I dreaded telling my husband the truth."

The trip home was difficult as she shared her news and fear with her husband. A visit to see the doctor confirmed her intuition: Grace had breast cancer.

"I was diagnosed with breast cancer more than forty years ago. I kept it very private as we lived in a small town and no one really talked about breast cancer back then. The doctor told me that a radical mastectomy was my only option so that's what I did."

The surgery was very invasive. The surgeon removed Grace's chest wall muscle all of the way down to her ribs, all of her lymph nodes, and some of the veins in her arms.

"I felt like I had hit a brick wall when on I woke up from the mastectomy. It was a difficult recovery but I just took one day at a time."

The pathology report was grim and Grace was given a poor prognosis. She expected the same outcome as her mother and grandmother. Fear cast a shadow over Grace's outlook on life.

"At first, I didn't want to shop or buy anything for myself. I would look at a new outfit in the store and think 'I won't be around to wear that so why buy it?' It was such a challenge in the beginning but I tried to keep living a normal life."

Grace predicted her own survival based on the observation of her mother's battle with breast cancer. Her mom had survived six years after diagnosis, so Grace presumed that she would have the same amount of time. Faced with her own mortality, she made a decision that would impact the rest of her life.

"I made up my mind that I would make the best of my six years. I stayed busy and volunteered with Reach to Recovery. I would visit women who were in the hospital recovering from their mastectomy. I received much more from the program that I was able to give. It helped me heal."

As she healed physically, Grace slowly began to change her outlook for the future.

"I would look in the mirror and tell myself, 'Grace, stop feeling sorry for yourself. Others have it much worse than you do.' I took it one day at a time and then I would suddenly realize that I hadn't thought about breast cancer for a day, a week, and then a month. I thanked the good Lord for every day that He gave me."

As weeks turned into years, Grace tried to live life to the fullest but she was plagued with fears about recurrence. Panic crept in with every new ache or pain, often resulting in a visit to the doctor. The passage of time helped her learn to sort through those feelings and move past the fear.

"I leaned on my husband so much through the hard days. He was so compassionate and supportive. He always told me that I looked beautiful. I also leaned on my faith. I'm not deeply religious, but I gave myself to God and asked Him to help me through it."

As years turned into decades, Grace continued to appreciate every day. She was quick to reach out and help others who needed it. As breast cancer faded into her past, she looked at her experience differently.

"You don't ever forget it, but it gets easier. I looked at my life differently. I wouldn't change anything about my journey through breast cancer. It was a fight that I won. I used to celebrate every anniversary of my diagnosis, but it's been so long now. I acknowledge that date but no longer feel a need to celebrate since it is a part of my past."

Reflecting back on her life, Grace believes that breast cancer changed her in many ways.

"It made me appreciate things that I had taken for granted and helped me realize that some things just don't matter. There were times when I thought that maybe my life was coming to an end. It changes you but some of those changes are for the better."

She is proud of her accomplishments in life and is grateful for her family.

"I enjoyed many years with my husband. He passed away fifteen years ago which was very difficult. I miss him terribly but I cherish our time together."

Grace shares her insight into why she believes she has survived breast cancer for more than four decades and is still going strong.

"For some reason, God let me slip through a crack and live. I made a pact with Him that I would live each day as it comes. I tried to have a good attitude and go on with my life. I was thankful for each day and I appreciate how fortunate I am to have lived so long."

Looking to the future, Grace has done everything she set out to accomplish in life. She revels in her longevity.

"If someone would have told me that I would live to see the age of ninety-one, I would have said you're absolutely crazy. But here I am, after all of these years. The most exciting thing in my life has been to live long enough to meet my great-grandchildren. I never dreamed that I would live to see my grandchildren grow up. There is so much joy in being a great-grandma and holding my great-grandchildren! What more could I ever ask for out of life?"

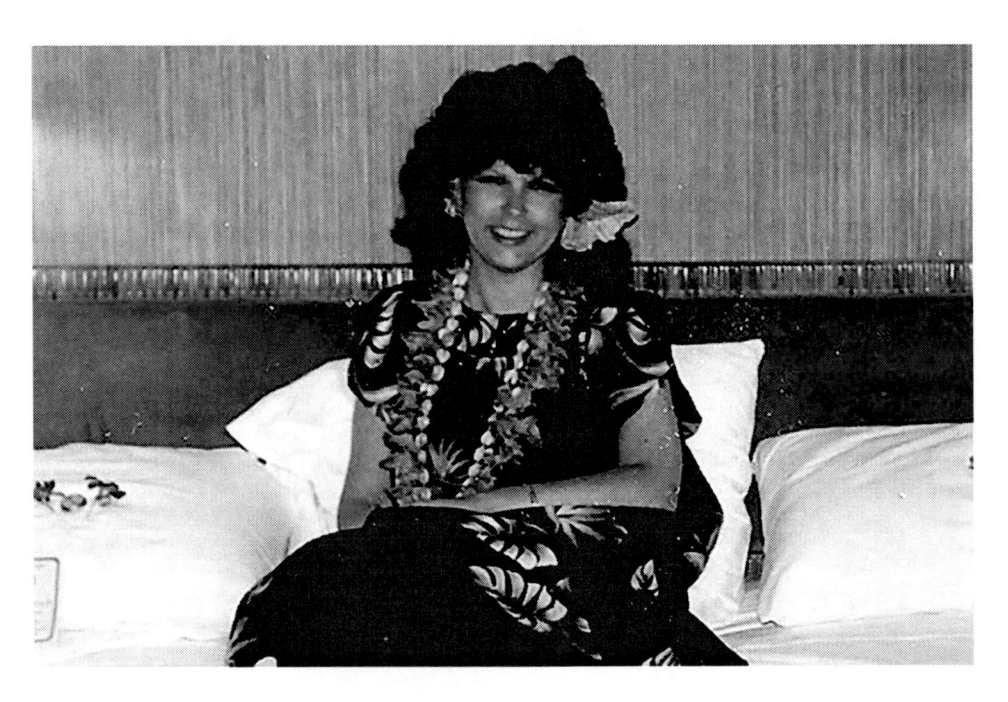

Marsha celebrating life after breast cancer in Hawaii one month after finishing chemotherapy.

CHAPTER 23 | Marsha Polys

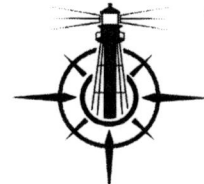

Celebrating Life Since She Was Diagnosed
in January 1986
St. Louis, MO

*"The doctor told everyone that I would not survive.
But no one told me. So, I kept on living."*

Marsha was enjoying life as a busy mom to three children, daughters in sixth and eighth grades and a ten-year-old son. She enjoyed her work at the local bank and spending time with her husband, family, and friends. Life was good when she developed pneumonia, which warranted a chest X-ray.

"The X-ray technician asked me if I had prosthetic breasts. I said no and she said that there must have been something on the film that caused a shadow. I didn't think much of it at the time."

Times were different nearly three decades ago. The "shadow" on the films was not further examined. Marsha went home and continued to battle pneumonia. Further testing failed to reveal a cause for her illness. The doctors grew more concerned when she lost twenty pounds without dieting.

The concept of a self-breast exam was just coming into vogue at the time. Marsha's unexplainable weight loss, combined with a self-exam culminated into a grim discovery. She found a lump on the bottom of her breast.

"Everyone kept telling me I was too young to have breast cancer. I was only thirty-six years old. They told me not to worry. I went to see my doctor, who sent me to a surgeon for X-rays. He was baffled by the results. Not only did I have breast cancer, but the tumor had fingers. Within two days, I was having a mastectomy."

The surgery took more than five hours due to the extensive amount of cancer in both her breast and lymph nodes. The doctor removed thirty-eight lymph nodes, twenty-four of which contained cancer. Marsha was still in recovery when the doctor met with her husband and sister-in-law. He shared unfathomable news: Marsha would not survive. They estimated that she would live three to six months at the most. The breast cancer was too aggressive and too advanced. Everyone in the family discussed the situation but no one told Marsha.

"I was prepared for the possibility of losing my breast because my doctor had warned me they would take the whole thing if it looked bad. I woke up and it was gone. I could accept losing my breast but everyone was crying. My mother-in-law, sister-in-law, even my husband. I had no idea that they had been given such terrible news."

Marsha's hospital room was full of flowers, cards, and music boxes. Her coworkers and customers from the bank were all praying for her and she was confident she would survive.

"I made a pact with God. I told Him that my husband couldn't raise our kids without me. I told Him He could take me later but not now."

As she began to heal from her surgery, Marsha's brother-in-law who was a doctor polled his colleagues to find the best cancer doctor in the area. He discovered an esteemed oncologist at a major hospital in St. Louis who would accept her case.

"My doctor is the person who saved my life. He was up to date on all of the research. I started a new type of chemotherapy not yet approved by insurance. I had to go inpatient for the first treatment and my body rejected it, so they had to put me under for the rest of the treatments. My dad would take me to my appointments so my husband could work. We never called it going to chemotherapy because it was so hard on my parents. We would say we were going for a blood test."

After her second chemotherapy treatment, Marsha went in for a full-body scan to see if the cancer was spreading. Once again, the news was grim. She had two spots on her spine and another one on her chest. The oncologist told her brother-in-law that the cancer had spread and that Marsha had less than three months to live. Once again, no one told Marsha that she would not survive.

"My husband went to Our Lady of Snows and purchased Lourdes water. He had the Sisters pray for me and he bathed those spots with Lourdes water every day. He believed that the Virgin Mary would heal me and he prayed to her constantly. Two weeks later they did another MRI and the spots had disappeared. Confused, the doctors ordered a bone biopsy which confirmed that the cancer was gone. My doctor told my brother-in-law that he didn't have a clue what happened. He would have staked his reputation that the cancer had spread and now it was gone. He started referring to me as his miracle patient."

Marsha continued with chemotherapy which was often postponed due her blood levels. The side effects of the chemotherapy were grueling at times, but she had the support of her family, many friends, and coworkers. Determined to make the best of a difficult situation, her sister-in-laws took Marsha shopping for wigs like they were shopping for a wedding dress. They bought different styles and colors to keep her spirits high. Once chemotherapy was finished, she went on a fabulous trip with her husband.

"My reward for finishing chemotherapy was a trip to Hawaii. I was still wearing a wig at the time. We planned the vacation halfway through my chemo treatments so I was really excited. We had so much fun on that trip. It was so beautiful and the people were so wonderful."

Radiation was not prescribed for Marsha. Her doctor informed her that the benefits would not outweigh the side effects due to her advanced cancer. He encouraged her to focus on her quality of life.

"He never told me that I wouldn't survive. All along, I had been thinking it would be a bad year but next year would be better. I told my husband, Larry, that he was worrying too much about me."

Larry was carrying a heavy burden with the knowledge that Marsha would not survive. It was heartbreaking to envision a future without his wife, but he had to be realistic. One day, he brought up a difficult subject that loomed near in the future, but Marsha remained oblivious.

"We were at the mall and Larry said that we had to talk about funerals, just in case. I told him that I wanted lots of flowers and then I asked him what he wanted at his funeral. I had no idea that he was actually preparing for my funeral."

Marsha recovered from her treatment and went back to work. She was unaware that word had spread that she was not going to survive.

"Apparently, everyone had written me off as dead and another woman wanted my job. I went in for a raise and they told me no. I found out later it was because they would have to pay out more for my death benefit. The bank was about to be sold and everyone was supposed to receive a $500 bonus, but my name wasn't on the list. I had no idea that they thought I would be dead by then. They had me in the grave and buried. I was so upset with everyone at my job because I had no idea what was going on. I kept telling them that they had taken my breast, not my brain. Back then, some people acted as though cancer was contagious and treated you as a leper. It was so frustrating."

Everyone had a fresh start when the bank sold, which was especially beneficial for Marsha. Her new boss didn't have any preconceived notions about her imminent demise. Determined to prove that she was an excellent employee, Marsha impressed everyone with her skills and hard work. She was rewarded with the very first computer and was promoted to a better job. She continued to heal physically and emotionally as one year led to another.

"I never missed my breast. I had a comfortable prosthetic bra and prosthesis. I had to be cancer free for at least five years before they would do reconstruction.

I had that surgery in 1990. They took the fat and muscle from my stomach for the surgery and I've been very happy with the results."

Over the years, Marsha was often the youngest woman in the waiting room at her oncology office. She has had a few scares but nothing like her first diagnosis.

"In 2008, I had a biopsy. It was just the very beginning of cancer, so I didn't need chemotherapy. My new doctor told me that I might have a recurrence in the future, but I shouldn't let it rule my life."

Reflecting back on her diagnosis, Marsha shares her insight about why she has survived breast cancer for nearly three decades and going strong.

"I firmly believe that my doctor's expertise, the Lourdes Water, green tea, and prayer saved my life. I have faith in the Virgin Mary and pray to her often. The combination of these things is what saved me."

Breast cancer brought many changes to Marsha's life.

"Before breast cancer, I was always in the background and definitely not assertive. I wasn't afraid to speak up after my diagnosis. It also taught me who my real friends were. I couldn't have survived without the support of those true friends and my family. I also learned that there is so much good in people. In a way, I'm glad it happened to me. It has given me the opportunity to help several friends make it through the challenge of battling cancer."

Marsha has enjoyed a wonderful life since her diagnosis. She has been back to Hawaii several times and she still enjoys the unwavering support of her husband.

"My husband has always been there for me. Over the years, he's had five heart attacks but he is still here. We are old now and we have a lifetime of memories."

Marsha feels blessed to have the opportunity to watch her children grow up and start families of their own.

"I'm lucky because my kids are happy and now I have grandchildren. They are the most wonderful things in the world. Being here for my kids' weddings and watching my grandchildren being born has been worth everything. I've had a good life and I'm happy."

Looking to the future, Marsha plans to enjoy spending quality time with her husband, her children, and her grandchildren.

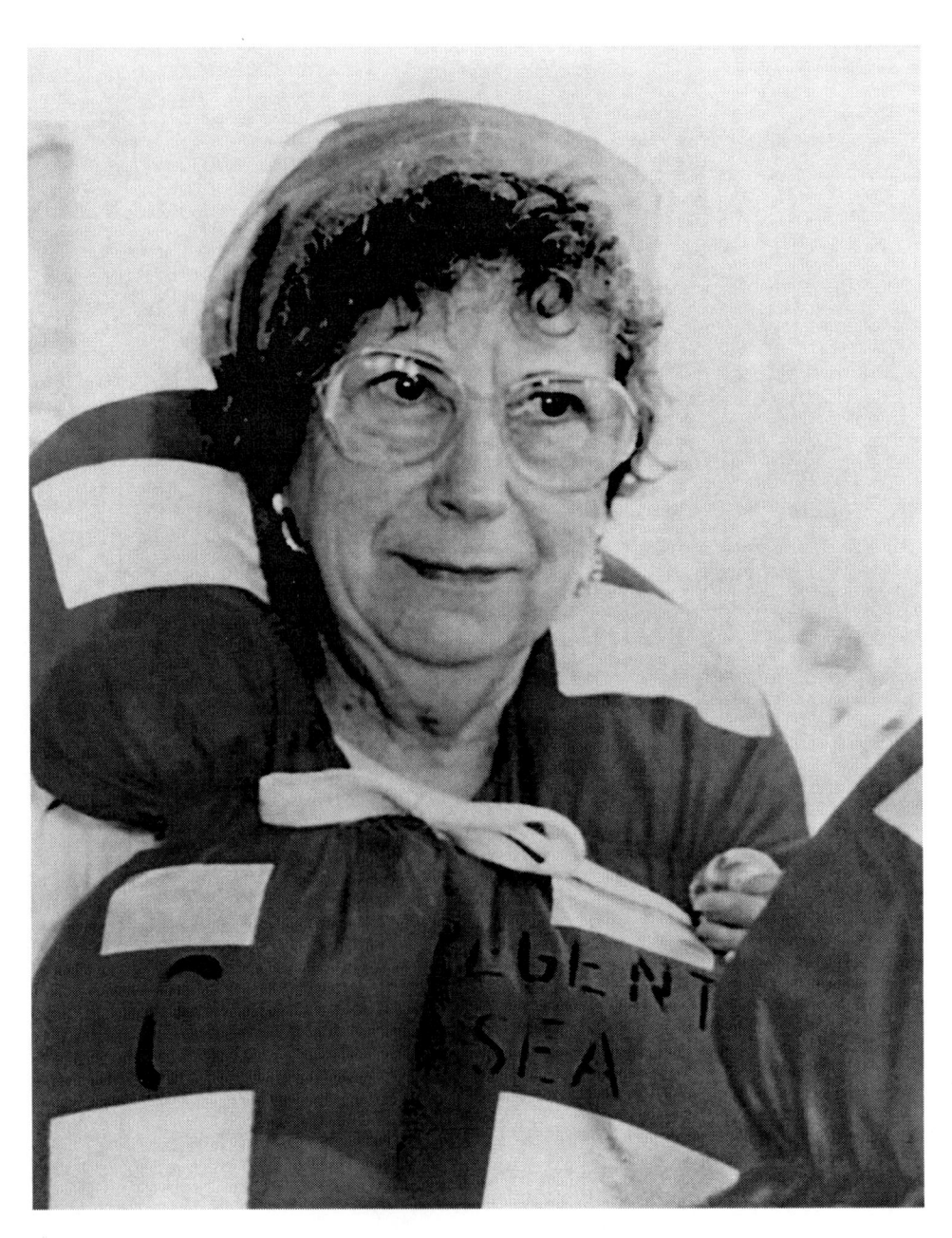

Francis celebrating life after breast cancer on a fun-filled cruise!

Chapter 24 | Francis Putney

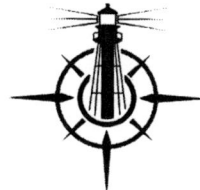

Celebrated Life for Forty-One Years
After Being Diagnosed in 1974
St. Louis, MO

"I decided that if it came back, the doctors would know how to handle it. I let it go. I don't really think about breast cancer anymore."

Francis was born in a time when breast cancer wasn't discussed . . . 1918 to be exact. She married a man who became a hero in World War II. A brave soldier who was captured in a photograph raising the flag on Hiroshima. Francis lived in the shadow of a legend, her husband, who was interviewed countless times throughout the years. She lived an ordinary life, proudly raising her two children and caring for her home.

Francis was fifty-seven when she became concerned about some unusual discharge from her right breast. Her husband rushed her to the doctor immediately.

"The doctor said that there was something there and the next thing I knew, he was cutting and sawing on me. They took everything on that side, even my rib. Times were different then. The doctors told you what to do and you did it, no questions asked. I feel bad for women now with all of these choices. It must be overwhelming to make all of those decisions. I was at the mercy of my doctor and he saved my life."

Recovering from surgery was not easy, requiring close to three weeks of recovery in the hospital. Her devoted husband was waiting to help her once she came home.

"My husband always says that the doctor did the cutting, but he did the curing. He put iodine on my incision every day so it would heal from the inside out. My skin grew back perfectly smooth."

Her doctor offered reconstruction but she didn't want to "mess with all of that." She wanted to heal and be done with breast cancer. The doctor did not offer any other type of treatment, so once she was healed from surgery, Francis got back to the business of life. She considers herself lucky after seeing others suffer with the side effects of treatment.

As she reflects back on her journey through breast cancer and her life at the age of ninety-six, Francis shares her thoughts as to why she has survived for more than forty-one years after diagnosis.

"I leaned heavily on my faith, which I still do today. So many women worry about the cancer coming back, but I never looked back. I decided that if it came back, the doctors would know how to handle it. I let it go. I don't really think about breast cancer anymore."

Francis has only one regret about her journey through breast cancer.

"I wish I would have stuck with physical therapy longer. My insurance ran out and I felt better, so I stopped both physical therapy and the exercises they told me to do to keep my arm strong. I still have pain under my arm today but it's a small price to pay."

Life after breast cancer has been wonderful for Francis and her family. Over the years, her family has grown to include four grandchildren and six great-grandchildren. Travels throughout the world with her husband include seven trips to Europe and a cruise to Alaska. One trip included a celebration during which they were deemed the King and Queen of Portugal for a day. Those many memories pale in comparison to a trip to Rome, where Francis was within inches of the pope.

"He was so close to me and we have great pictures. That was a really great day!"

Looking to the future, Francis plans to enjoy many more days with her husband, children, grandchildren, and great-grandchildren.

Update from the author: *It is with great sadness that I must share that Francis passed away on March 1, 2015. She was ninety-seven years old at the time. She left this world surrounded by her loving family. She lived a wonderful life with her husband, children, grandchildren, and great-grandchildren for forty-one years after being diagnosed with breast cancer. She is an inspiration to us all. Until we meet again, Francis! Thanks for the inspiration!*

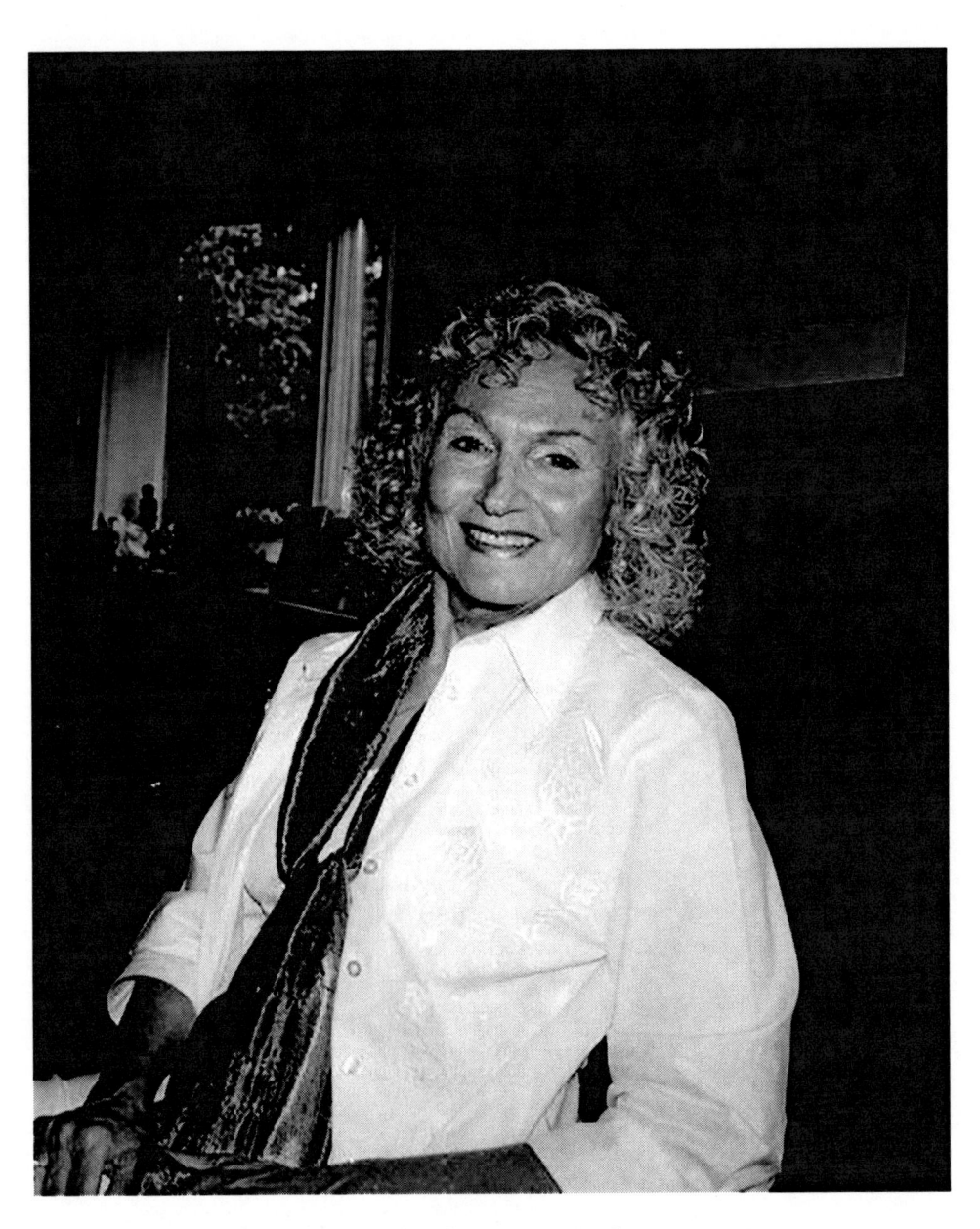

Gail celebrating life thirty years after breast cancer!

CHAPTER 25 | Gail Plude

Celebrating Life Since She Was Diagnosed
in May 1985
Fairfield, CT

"God answered my prayers for healing and in addition blessed me with a loving husband. My hope is that other women who are going through breast cancer will benefit from my experience, especially single women who fear they are unlovable."

Gail had struggled with a challenging year of loss. A single mom to her ten-year-old daughter, she was still reeling from the unexpected death of her brother. One year prior, at the age of thirty-nine, he was diagnosed with a rare blood cancer and lost his battle within six weeks. Gail had recently connected to a new church just before his diagnosis and leaned heavily on her new friends at church to cope with her loss.

"I was traumatized by my brother's death and I spent the whole year afterwards growing my faith in my new church. I was spending time with my new Christian friends and went with them to a Billy Graham concert. That was the day that I accepted Jesus Christ as my Lord and Savior."

Three weeks later, Gail found a lump in her breast. Her fears were compounded by the many family members who had lost their battle with cancer throughout the years, including her grandmother, mother, father, aunt, and most recently, her brother. School was out the day of Gail's appointment, so she brought her daughter to the appointment. Shock set in as her doctor shared grim news. The lump was likely breast cancer and she needed a biopsy.

Shortly after the biopsy, Gail was devastated to hear the results of the pathology report. Her worst fears were confirmed . . . she had breast cancer.

"I thought it was a death sentence at the age of forty-three and that I wouldn't be around to raise my daughter. My doctor tried to reassure me by telling me that I had a ninety percent chance of surviving but I didn't believe him. They had told my brother the same thing and he died within six weeks of his diagnosis. I was terrified until about a week before surgery. I heard a sermon at church and saw God working through my breast cancer journey. My faith helped me through my surgery and treatment."

Gail had a successful lumpectomy followed by radiation. Her new Christian friends visited often during her treatment. They listened to her fears, encouraged her, and helped her in her walk of faith.

"I had been a single parent for eleven years. I had a young daughter and now I had been diagnosed with breast cancer. I was afraid that no man would ever want me. I tried to focus on my gratitude for being alive and at some point, I accepted that I would never have a man in my life."

A month later, a new young man joined Gail's church. He showed in an interest in Gail but she was still having radiation. She summoned all of her courage to share the truth that would surely send him running in the other direction.

"I was so nervous to tell him that I had breast cancer but I couldn't start a relationship with him until he knew the truth. I told him that I was in the middle of radiation for breast cancer and he told me that he already knew about my diagnosis. I was in shock. He knew the truth and still wanted to get to know me. I knew in that moment that God had brought us together."

The couple started dating and then got married quickly. All of Gail's fears about being single forever were alleviated and she found true happiness and acceptance in her new husband.

"I have seen God working in my life and others. He answered my prayers with my husband, who loves me, my daughter, my home, and my dog. I was really, really grateful. My hope is that single women who are going through breast cancer will be encouraged from my experience."

Gail healed physically and emotionally from her journey through breast cancer treatment. She is grateful to never have had a recurrence but she has had a few scares along the way. She had a mammogram with concerning results not long after she finished radiation.

"I prayed and prayed that it wasn't cancer. I panicked for about fifteen minutes then a peace came over me with an acceptance for whatever the diagnosis might be. I was so relieved when I got the call that it was just scar tissue."

She had regular mammograms for the next twenty-eight years, but they never cease to cause fear and anxiety. Gail uses prayer to overcome her fear every year. Two years ago, she had another scare with an inconclusive mammogram. She had a needle biopsy and lumpectomy but ultimately, she learned that it was just scar tissue.

"Here I am thirty years later! I'm seventy-two years old but I feel young. Breast cancer was a big part of my life but it was just a part of my whole life story. God has brought me this far."

Gail's positive outlook on life has inspired her to write about recovering from breast cancer and divorce. She has an incredible social media following where she tweets about faith, politics, and divorce.

"God has given me the platform to reach out and change the world back to the way it used to be. I try to make a difference in the world by tweeting about recovering from divorce and my view on politics and Christianity."

Gail's little girl is all grown up now and brings great joy to her mom. "My daughter is an amazing woman. I'm so thankful that she lives close so I can spend time with my grandsons. It is great fun to be a grandparent."

Gail celebrates her triumph over breast cancer every May. She offers reassurance to anyone who has gone through breast cancer treatment that it gets better with time. Reflecting back over her life, she shares her insight as to why she has survived breast cancer for thirty years.

"I believe that I have survived for so long because of my faith. Fear has been replaced by faith as I have watched the beauty of God work through it all."

Looking to the future, Gail plans to have fun every day and help her grandchildren become the best people they can be. Now that she is retired, she has recently taken on a new endeavor. She had always been terrified to get onto a boat, but her husband loves to fish for salmon, bass, and bluefish. Determined to overcome her fear, Gail took a class to learn how to drive the boat so they can enjoy the water together.

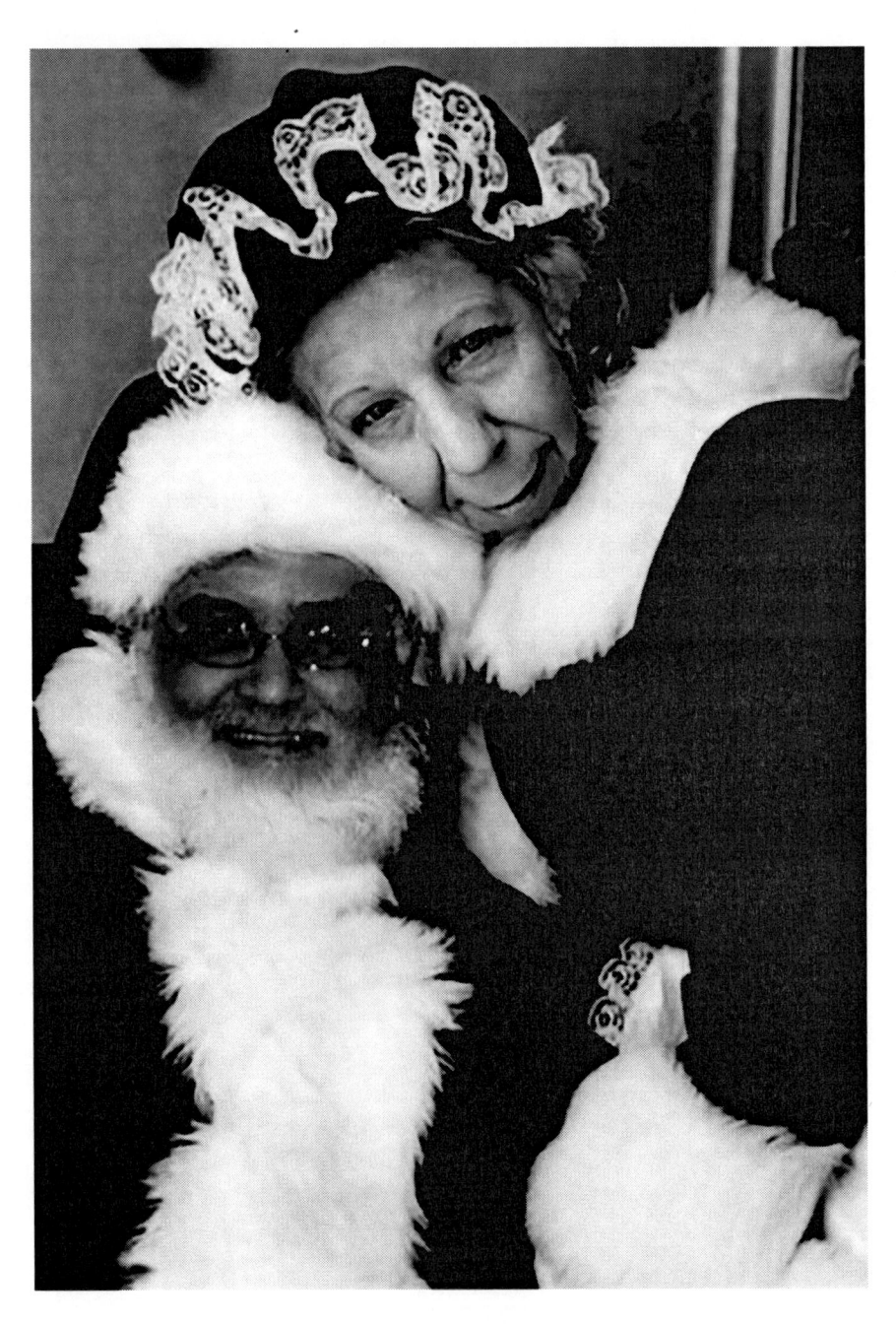

May celebrating life after breast cancer as Mrs. Claus!

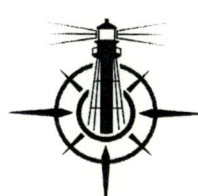

CHAPTER 26 | May Ne

Celebrating Life Since She Was Diagnosed
in October 1986
Abita Springs, LA

"I never had a bit of fear due to the peace that came from a prayer that I wrote early on the morning of my surgery. I went into that operating room with a sense of peace all around me."

Strength and resilience have been a common theme throughout May's life. Plagued by cancer throughout her family, she had lost six siblings, both parents, and her first husband to the disease. Perhaps most difficult was watching her youngest son battle childhood leukemia. Through all of these challenges, May leaned on her faith and stayed strong for her children and stepchildren. Her positive outlook on life was bolstered by a new love. Still a newlywed, May wasn't overly concerned when she discovered a lump in her breast.

"I had a ten-year history of fibrocystic disease so I wasn't worried. I went to see a surgeon for a biopsy but there wasn't any fluid in the lump. They sent me back for a mammogram but it was too hard to read it because of the inflammation from the biopsy. I had to wait to do a surgical biopsy."

May was recovering in the hospital when the doctors shared their shocking discovery. She had breast cancer. A mastectomy was scheduled within two weeks. Always the optimist, May found a way to process this new turn of events in her life.

"I never had a bit of fear due to the peace that came from a prayer that I wrote early on the morning of my surgery. I went into that operating room with a sense of peace all around me."

The pathology report held grim news. The cancer had spread to her lymph nodes. Reconstruction was very new at the time so May's doctors advised against it, due to her family history. After healing from surgery, May entered the next phase of treatment: six months of chemotherapy.

"I never questioned God but I did wonder why all of my siblings had some form of cancer, as did my mom and my son. I found that in some ways, it was easier to be the patient after having been a caregiver for so many loved ones. The doctors were able to give me medicine for my side effects but caregivers aren't given anything to cope with the fear and guilt."

of May's biggest concerns about chemotherapy was losing her hair. Her ~~~s told her that hair loss was inevitable so May leaned on her faith.

"I said, 'Lord, I realize that I have to do this. Please, take the boob but don't take my hair.' I lost every hair on my body but not on my head. To this day, all I can say is 'Thank you, Jesus!'"

While she felt blessed to keep her hair, May struggled with other side effects of chemotherapy. Even on her worse days, she never stopped enjoying life.

"I wanted to go see my sister-in-law in California. The doctor told me no but I went anyway. I slept in the trunk with the backseat folded down on the way. We had to stop in Mexico for blood work because I was so sick but I had so much fun! We saw Vegas and snow on Mount Summit."

As the holidays approached, May's spunky attitude and zest for life clashed with her doctor's advice.

"My doctor told me not to prepare Christmas dinner. My husband just looked at him and said 'Give it up, doc.' I prepared everyone's favorite dish even though I was sick. It was a great dinner."

At one point, the side effects of chemotherapy warranted an admission to the hospital. It was during this hospital stay that her youngest son, now in remission from childhood leukemia, received the phone call everyone had been anticipating. He was granted his "wish" through a childhood cancer foundation.

"My son was twelve at the time and had always wanted to go see the band Alabama. I left the hospital to get his wish granted. We rode in a limo and met the band members. My son wanted McDonald's for dinner so we took the limo through the drive-through. It truly was a night to remember."

Life went on after May finished chemotherapy. Always the optimist and determined to help others, May found a job that put a smile on the faces of children during the holiday season.

"One year, I got a job as Mrs. Claus which was just the best job in the world. Seeing all of those children smile with the magic of Christmas was so much fun."

Always embracing life, May loves joining the festivities of Mardi Gras in New Orleans.

"I love dressing in my pink boa and dancing in the streets with everyone. I am just a crazy Cajun lady who loves life!"

She has offered support to countless women who have been touched by breast cancer, often sharing the prayer that she wrote so many years ago:

> *John 11:4. "This sickness is not unto death, but for the Glory of God. That the son of God may be Glorified by it."*

May's Prayer:

Take this sickness in my life and use it and me, Lord, for your Glory, oh God. Make me strong, Lord, so that I can face the days to come. Lord, I want to be strong, I want to show the world that with Your help and Your wisdom that this illness, this cancer can and will be healed and used to Glorify your name, Lord. Let the Holy Spirit fill me so I do not feel any emptiness from the surgery. Help me to face the days to come with pride in my heart and in my soul for You, Lord, so the flesh will mean little to me. I know, Lord, as long as I have You in me and to walk with me, I can do this. Use me, Lord, to show others as long as they have You and The Holy Spirit within them, that they need not miss any parts that man can take from them. In Jesus' name I pray, Amen.

While breast cancer was challenging for May, it deepened her faith which helped her cope with the loss of her second husband twenty-four years after her diagnosis. She later met her soul mate, Carey.

"I looked beyond the fact that Carey was a quadriplegic. He always had a smile on his face and something sweet to say. He taught me more in the year and a half that we were together than anyone ever had before. He was phenomenal. It was heartbreaking when he suddenly passed away. I have missed him dearly."

Reflecting back over the last twenty nine years, May shares her insight as to why she has survived breast cancer for nearly three decades and is still going strong.

"God is in charge and I'm blessed to have a good relationship with the Lord. I also had a positive attitude. I needed the doctors but my positive attitude made all of the difference."

Every year, May has celebrated the anniversary of her diagnosis. She has combined her cancer anniversary with her bucket list, checking off one item every October.

"I have had so much fun on my 'Celebration of Life' day! One year I went to see the Chippendale dancers which was a night to remember! Another year, I was serenaded by a jazz group with my sister-in-law. There are so many memories over the years! Life is too short. We need to enjoy it while we can!"

Looking to the future, one of her most anticipated items on her bucket list is to ride in a convertible with the top down and the radio up. She hopes to finish her book, *Both Sides of the Fence*, which shares the challenges of being a patient and a caregiver. Most importantly, she looks forward to enjoying her children and stepchildren in years to come.

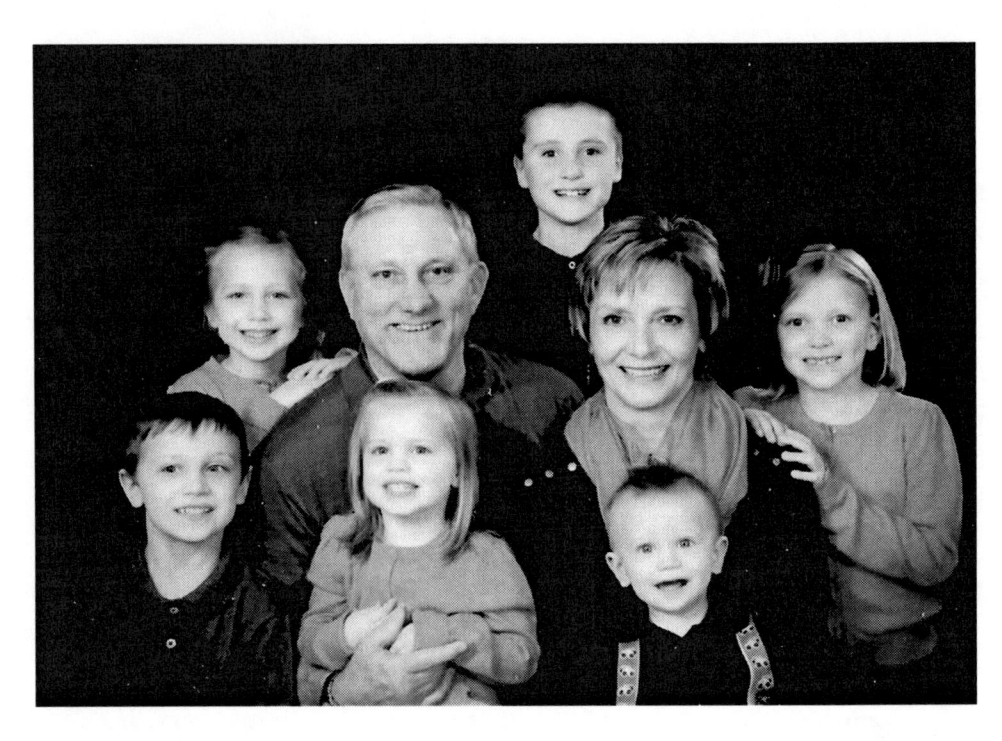

Sherry celebrating life after breast cancer with her husband and grandchildren!

CHAPTER 27 | Sherry Suon

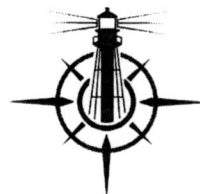

Celebrating Life Since She Was Diagnosed
in July 1991
Wauseon, OH

"When my treatments were done and my 'grounding' days had subsided, I had one day of sick leave left. That was a true God Sighting for me."

Camping, family trips, laughter, and love all describe Sherry's life with her husband, thirteen-year-old son, and eleven-year-old daughter back in 1991. Working at the local high school offered a deep satisfaction in addition to the family's involvement with their church and community. Discovering a lump in her breast wasn't overly alarming. Sherry was only thirty-five and had a clean mammogram just a few months prior. A trip to the doctor resulted in reassurance that she did not need to be concerned. However, the discovery of a mirror-image lump in her other breast prompted a needle aspiration on both lumps.

Sherry was enjoying the quiet calm of a school building during summer break when she received the call from her doctor's office. Still confident that all was fine, the nurse's request to meet the doctor at the hospital did not set off any alarms.

"I never processed the idea that it might be bad news. I thought I was just going to talk to my doctor. He told me that I had breast cancer. I was so stunned that I felt like he was talking about someone else. I found myself in same-day surgery, having a lumpectomy on one breast and a biopsy on the other. I kept thinking that I was healthy and active. How could I possibly have breast cancer?"

Sherry made the call that would change her parents' life, sharing her difficult news. Always supportive, they barely took time to pack before driving five hundred miles to be with their daughter in her time of need.

"Seeing my mom's face as she walked up the drive was heartbreaking. Mom kept saying that it should be her that was sick, not me. God's timing was so good. Mom had retired several years earlier and dad had retired two months prior, allowing them the time to stay with us to help so much."

The pathology report from the lumpectomy prompted the need for a lymph node dissection the following week. More grim news followed. The breast cancer had spread to one of twenty-seven lymph nodes. Sherry's pastor offered reassurance that that she had done nothing wrong. That message set the tone for Sherry to begin healing.

In the meantime, Sherry and her husband had to break the news to their children.

"The fear in my kids' eyes was heart wrenching. My son held it all in while he processed the information. My daughter and my husband sobbed. When my husband's handkerchief wasn't doing the job, the kids got a bath towel to help dry all of his tears. I have such a distinct memory of that day all of these years later."

Daily radiation treatments brought only mild side effects, but the forty-five-minute drive each way was taxing. One week into treatment, Sherry asked for help from friends and family to act as a chauffeur for the long drive. She kept working throughout the radiation regimen, celebrating her last radiation and her thirty-sixth birthday with a nice lunch with her husband.

Two weeks later, Sherry's doctor surgically implanted a Hickman catheter. This would aid in the administration of chemotherapy.

"My doctor put me on a heavy regimen of chemotherapy. He told me he was bringing out the big guns."

Over the next four months, Sherry's schedule was dictated by her chemotherapy infusions. One week included a trip to her oncologist's office for a three-hour intravenous drip. The following week Sherry's treatment became mobile for three straight days, administered through her Hickman catheter.

"My husband would play Scrabble with me to pass the time during my three-hour chemotherapy treatments. It was hard on him, too. One day, as the nurse was connecting the IV to my catheter, he got teary eyed and told me he wished that they could give him the drugs that day. God made sure one of us was strong when the other was not."

One of the most anticipated days for children throughout the world, Christmas Eve, was filled with bittersweet emotions that year. Standing in front of the mirror with her husband watching, Sherry's hair fell out with the slightest tug. Tears streamed down their faces but once she was done, they dried their tears and joined their children, determined to enjoy the holiday. Sherry enjoyed her new look in the safety of her home, trying on scarves and allowing the kids to rub her bald head. But everyone knew to watch out if the doorbell rang. Sherry would run frantically for her wig.

"I would run around yelling, 'Where's my hair?' because I never wanted anyone to see me without it. But I was blessed that I wore my wig during the winter months and never had to deal with the weather being too hot. However, the Northwest Ohio winds were definitely an issue. My husband would call me to announce that it was a 'wig warning day' on really windy days. He was always good at keeping a smile on my face."

Chemotherapy and baldness never stopped Sherry from working, but her role at her children's school presented a unique challenge. She was determined to avoid the embarrassment of her children being labeled as having a "sick mom." Her coworkers renewed her faith in society when they approached the payroll department, requesting permission to share their sick days with Sherry.

"These co-workers often gave the impression of being rough and tough people but deep inside, they were the most considerate. When my treatments were done and my 'grounding' days had subsided, I had *one* day of sick leave left. That was a true God Sighting for me. I believe that God will always provide just the amount that you can deal with, providing just the amount that you need."

Although she continued to work, chemotherapy often caused Sherry's blood count to drop. Her doctor advised her to stay home and away from people to avoid germs throughout her treatment.

"My kids always had a good laugh on those days, referring to them as 'mom is grounded' days. Again, keeping the joy in the house is very important, even during the struggles."

The outpouring of support from the community was overwhelming at times. Cards filled her mailbox and remain packed away in a special place more than two decades later. Perhaps most touching was the support offered to her husband at his local business.

"It was such a relief to me when they asked my husband how he was doing. The men in church were all so supportive. Breast cancer is hard on the entire family which was something that we had never considered in the past. Now, we try to comfort others who are going through any kind of tragedy. I think we go through things so that we can help others."

Sherry finished treatment just in time for the annual family camping trip. Bravery was overcome with panic as she decided to leave her wig behind, debuting her stubble of hair.

"As we drove further from home, I started sobbing. I wanted my wig. Everyone was comforting me and my kids were telling me that I could do it. I did it and I never wore my wig again. I started the next school year with very short hair."

Sherry experienced one of her lowest points after treatment ended. After nine months of constant attention and reassurance, she bid her nurses farewell.

"How do so many breast cancer survivors cope with overwhelming emotions and fear as they face life after breast cancer? I leaned on my faith and my husband. It took a lot of prayer and time to move past it."

Sherry lives her faith in her community, as well. She offers support to anyone who is facing a crisis, calling her random encounters "divine appointments." She studies the Bible when she is struggling and searches for "God Sightings" in her daily walk. Over the years, she shares those events with her kids when tucking them in at night.

"There was a point in my life that I was complacent about my faith. Breast cancer shook me and helped me care more about others and my faith."

Sherry had several scares and many biopsies throughout the last twenty-four years but has never had a recurrence. She can empathize with other breast cancer survivors who are paralyzed with the fear of recurrence years after a breast cancer diagnosis.

"I recently had neck problems. Subconsciously, I was afraid that it was cancer, even all of these years later. I went to the doctor in a panic. He told me that I was fine and that I just needed to move my neck. He ordered a bone scan for my mental health because I didn't need it physically. He called me with good results and I fell apart and cried. I felt better emotionally and then I was able to move my neck. It's really hard to move past the fear but it's a normal part of the process."

Sherry's biggest cheerleaders during her treatment are all grown up now. Both her son and daughter live close which allows her to spoil her six grandchildren, three boys and three girls. She has enjoyed marvelous vacations with her family including a trip to Disneyland with her daughter's family.

"I felt like a kid again. I thought my roller coaster days were over but I was always the first in line. I love being a grammy to my grandchildren and try to live my faith in front of them."

Looking back over nearly a quarter of a century, Sherry shares her insight as to why she has survived breast cancer for twenty-four years and counting.

"I think God has a bigger plan and He has something He wants me to do. My faith played such an important role in my journey through breast cancer and still does today."

Sherry is looking forward to a new phase of life in the near future.

"Retirement is dangling like a carrot in front of us. I look forward to spending more time with my children and grandchildren. My husband wants to go to Italy for our forty-year anniversary. I also think it would be great fun to go parasailing and ride in a fighter jet, both of which are on my bucket list."

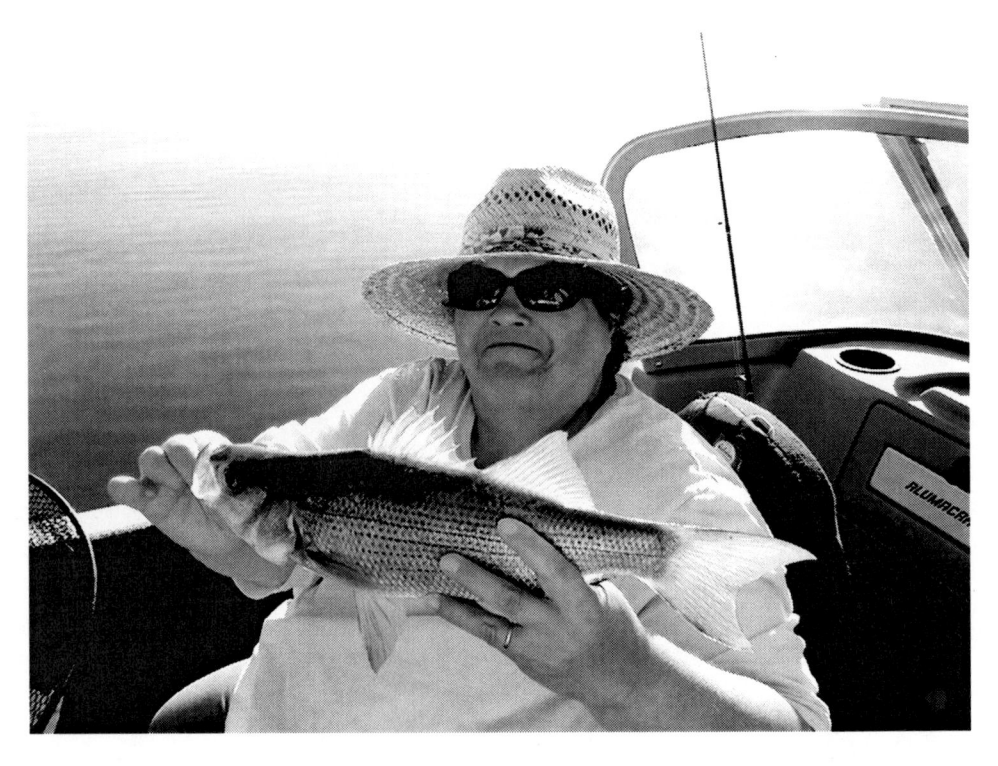

Carol celebrating life after breast cancer fishing with her late husband at Bull Shoals Lake!

Chapter 28 | Carol Smith

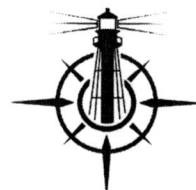

Celebrating Life Since She Was Diagnosed
in 1985
Fenton, MO

"Shortly after surgery, my husband wanted to buy me a beautiful new coat. I didn't think I would be alive long enough to wear it but he bought it anyway. I wouldn't have made it without him."

Scarred at a young age by a host of relatives battling breast cancer, Carol was religious with self-breast exams from a young age. Her mother had been diagnosed at the age of thirty-three with metastatic breast cancer which prompted Carol to schedule her first baseline mammogram at the same age. Fear set in when the doctor discovered a suspicious lump and ordered a biopsy. Her prayers were answered when the pathology came back as benign.

Life went back to normal for a year until the next routine mammogram.

"My doctor walked in after my mammogram and told me that they had found a suspicious area in my breast. He hesitated and then admitted something that was just unbelievable. He had left a foreign object in my breast during my last surgery. It turned out to be a piece of tubing, which I had felt, but assumed was scar tissue. Sadly, that was the least of my worries. I was lying in the hospital bed, recovering from surgery when they told me that I had breast cancer. The image of my aunt, who had passed away from breast cancer came into my mind and I started to cry."

The onslaught of foreign oncology terminology was overwhelming and this was well before the time of Google, so Carol drove her young children, ages four and eleven, to the library to research her diagnosis and treatment options.

"I had Stage III Infiltrating Intraductal Carcinoma and lymph node involvement. I told my doctor that I wanted a mastectomy. I was prepared to do chemotherapy, radiation . . . whatever it took to survive. I was stunned when my primary care physician told me that I shouldn't have chemo because I would lose my hair. I didn't care about my hair. I only wanted to live so that I could raise my children."

Carol's husband was her first and only true love of her life. They started dating at the age of sixteen and were married just after graduating from high school.

He was her rock throughout treatment. He comforted her after her modified radical mastectomy when the fear and anxiety were at their worst.

"I thought that I was a goner because of my aunt. Shortly after surgery, my husband wanted to buy me a beautiful new coat. I didn't think I would be alive long enough to wear it but he bought it anyway. One night, lying in bed, the thought washed over me, 'I could die.' My husband held me while I cried. His next words changed everything, 'You're not going to die, Carol. I guarantee it.' I believed him and I never felt that way again. I wouldn't have made it without him."

Six chemotherapy treatments were the next course of action. Carol struggled with severe illness after each treatment but she never lost her hair. She finished her journey through treatment with a prophylactic mastectomy on the other side, which left her husband balancing work, the children, and the household.

"My husband brought the kids to see me in the hospital. I asked them what they had for dinner and they told me pot pies several nights in a row. I looked at my husband and he told me not to worry, they were different flavors of pot pies every night. He was such a wonderful husband and father, but he wasn't into cooking and cleaning. I got home from the hospital and my floors were so dirty. I was tired of lying around, so I got down on my knees and scrubbed the entire floor with my good arm. It made me so happy to have a clean house and to be back to normal."

Carol became an advocate in her own way after recovery from treatment. She visited other women in the hospital with Reach to Recovery for five years. The local newspaper wrote a story featuring her journey through breast cancer, promoting mammograms and self-exams which led to her offering comfort to countless others throughout the years.

"I was outraged when reading an article in the local paper about a woman who said that she could never live without her breasts. I had to do something, because I knew women would lose their lives if they believed this woman. I wrote a letter to the editor in an effort to balance her opinion."

Breast cancer continued to plague Carol's family. While her mother had made a full recovery and survived for thirty-nine years after her diagnosis with metastatic cancer, other family members were not as fortunate. Her cousin battled the disease in her early forties and that cousin's daughter was only twenty-three when she was diagnosed. It was time to do something as a family. Everyone had tested negative for the BRCA1 and BRCA2 gene but there had to be a genetic component. An article in *St. Louis Magazine* led Carol's family to a researcher/oncologist who is studying new breast cancer genes. Everyone in the family rolled up their sleeves to donate blood for a targeted study in her family. Time will tell, but everyone is hopeful that this study will lead to new insight into the genetic component of breast cancer. Carol is very excited to be a part of helping others by participating in this study.

"Ten of us have fought breast cancer: my mom, sister, aunt, niece, five cousins, and me. Two of my brothers are fighting other kinds of cancer. There is a genetic link and someday, we will find it."

Carol has enjoyed a wonderful life since her breast cancer diagnosis thirty years ago. She raised her children and started a career after they left home. She feels blessed to have enjoyed forty-three years of marriage to her true love, her loving and devoted husband who passed away in 2011.

"I will miss my husband until the day I take my last breath, but I am so blessed to have lived this long. When I was first diagnosed, I remember praying, 'Please God, let me live to see my kids raised.' He's done that and I am so thankful. My life was not overly exciting but we have a lifetime of great memories."

Family trips hold a special place in Carol's heart, but her most exciting trip came about when she was only nineteen.

"I had married my first and only love in July of 1969. He left for Vietnam the next month, so we never had a honeymoon. The military arranged for a week of rest and relaxation for him in Hawaii and I had the opportunity to fly over to see him. I had never traveled or been on a plane, so I was terrified. But the moment when he walked off of that plane in Hawaii was indescribable. We spent five days enjoying Hawaii for our honeymoon."

Reflecting back on her journey through breast cancer, Carol shares her insights into why she survived the disease for nearly three decades.

"I couldn't have made it without my husband. But it also helped that I always tried to stay positive and I was determined to move past treatment. My doctors were great but most importantly, my faith has helped me through all of it. Breast cancer led me back to church. I wasn't a believer when I was diagnosed but God was seeking me. I found a new church during treatment and was saved during a service. I know that when I take my last breath, I will go to Heaven."

Looking to the future, Carol plans to spend many years spoiling her grandchildren and enjoying her children. She lives with her son and his family, which allows Carol to spoil her young grandson on a daily basis. Her daughter and her husband live nearby, along with her other grandson.

"I have done a lot in my life, experienced true love and have a great family. I wouldn't change a thing."

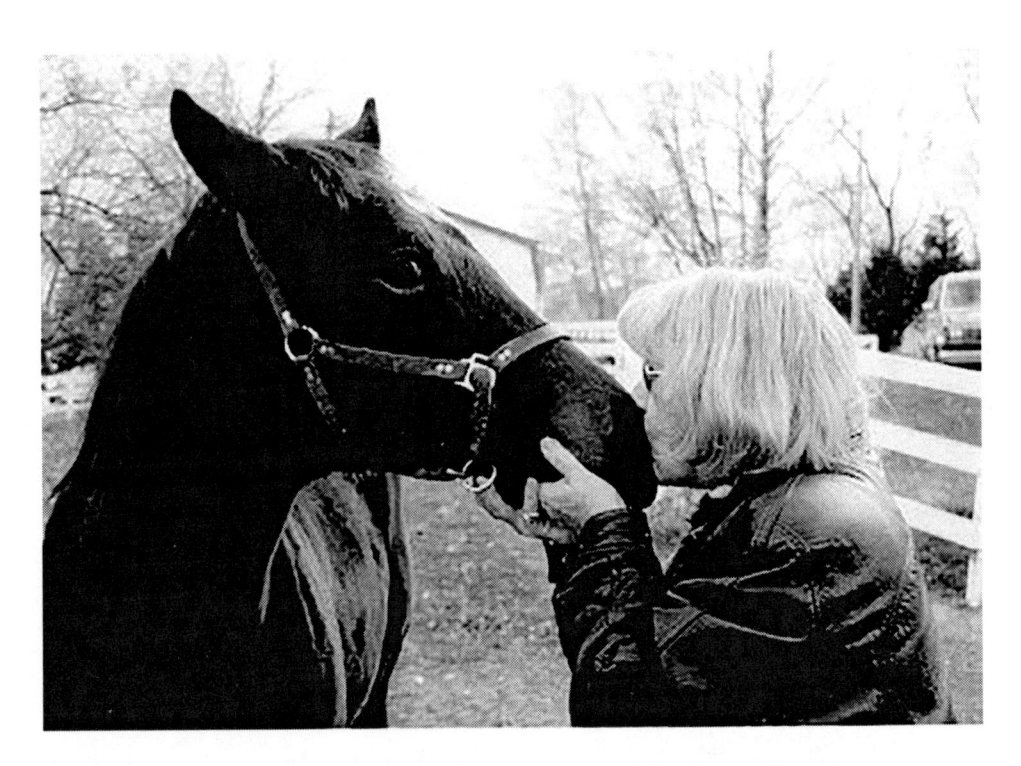

Patti celebrating life after breast cancer with her beloved horse!

Chapter 29 | Patti Nacci

Celebrating Life Since She Was Diagnosed
in November 1980
Fairview Heights, IL

"I said no to chemotherapy and radiation. I put myself in the hands of my Lord. I knew that I would live if He wanted me to live."

Patti was loving life, newly married to a wonderful man who shared her passion for horses. Normally very healthy, she had been struggling with severe headaches. Everything changed one morning in a hotel room on a trip to race horses. As she bent over the sink to brush her teeth, she noticed an indentation in her breast. Her hands moved across her breast and she made a discovery that flooded her body with fear. Unwilling to ruin the trip, she kept her discovery a secret until another debilitating headache caused her to miss the races. She shared her frightening news with her husband on the way home.

Patti's job provided great connections at a local hospital. Her new doctor initially thought the lump was a cyst, but called her later in the day to deliver the news that would shake her to the core: she had cancer and needed surgery.

"My first thoughts were, 'I'm dead.' I banged my head against the wall and cried. I walked back to my office to call my husband."

Patti had a radical mastectomy and lymph node surgery. She was not interested in reconstruction because she did not feel that her breasts made her a woman. She knew that her husband, Vince, felt the same way but his way of helping her cope with her loss is one that still moves her to tears.

"Vince asked to see my incision the day after surgery. I turned away as he gently took my arm out of the sling and opened my gown. He reached down and kissed my bandaged incision. I'll never forget his words: 'It's over now. We can move on.' He was so supportive. I knew that I couldn't lose with him by my side."

Vince wasn't the only one who helped Patti heal while in the hospital. A Reach to Recovery volunteer shared her story of healing and strength, which gave Patti courage.

"My volunteer was so great. She had an amazing outlook on life. She told me her tennis game was better than ever and reminded me that my breasts are not me, my soul is me. I still have that little bag from the American Cancer Society that she brought that day."

The day came for Patti to be discharged and she begged her husband to stop by the farm where they boarded their horse. Vince carefully assisted her out of the car and over to the fence. Patti called her horse through her tears and he came running through the pasture to greet her. She was so moved by what happened next that she sheds tears of joy to this day.

"I couldn't stop crying as I hugged my horse and kissed his muzzle. I kept telling him how much I loved him. He opened his mouth and licked my tears from my cheeks. It was my moment of healing. I knew in that moment that I would live. I thanked the Lord for the gifts He had given me . . . this man and this horse who loved me."

The couple's shared passion for horses shine through in the wedding picture, which includes Patti, Vince, and their horse in the background. She continued to heal with the help of her horse and her husband, especially as she was faced with tough decisions about treatment.

The pathology report was less than favorable. The cancer had spread to two of her lymph nodes which led her doctor to recommend chemotherapy and radiation. Patti had watched two cousins go through chemotherapy and radiation and not survive, while another aunt had only surgery and went on to live until the age of eighty-one. After much prayer, she shocked the doctor with her decision about treatment.

"I said no to chemotherapy and radiation. I put myself in the hands of my Lord. I knew that I would live if He wanted me to live. I was aware that the survival rate was about five years. My decisions were totally spiritual and not for everyone."

She continued to heal physically and emotionally. She never had another one of her debilitating headaches after surgery. One year later, Patti discovered that the farm where she boarded her horses was for sale. She desperately wanted to buy the ten acres of paradise but it was a stretch.

"We didn't have the money to buy the farm and Vince is a city boy from Philadelphia. He asked me what he would do with a farm if something happened to me. I told him he could sell it but in the meantime, let me enjoy it. We borrowed money for a down payment and bought the farm on bond to deed. Horses are the love of my life so buying the farm was a dream come true."

Patti's determination led her to buy another horse with an insurance payout for hail damage on a car. She bought a crippled thoroughbred who gave birth to two baby foals. She has owned and boarded many horses throughout the years. It wasn't always easy balancing her work schedule and the many hours that horses require every day, but Patti's heart was full of love and gratitude. She still lives on the farm today, with horses running around in the pasture behind the house.

"I've been blessed by my heavenly Father. I thank Him every day for my beautiful, beautiful life with my husband, my horses, and my rescued dogs."

Patti retired from the university after thirty-eight years of dedication and hard work. She enjoys spending more time at the farm, and several odd jobs to keep her busy. She worked part time in a western store and several department stores until she found a new niche. She started working as a caregiver to people who need in-home care.

"I love working with people who need me. I felt like I needed more training, so I went back to school at the age of seventy-five to become a certified nursing assistant. I am very selective with my cases and only work a couple of days per week, but I love making a difference."

Most recently, Patti returned to the university. She is working part time for her former chairman who is now ninety years old. She plans to continue working for the duration.

Patti also took up piano lessons and purchased a baby grand piano after retirement. She enjoys playing piano and is still taking lessons today. Breast cancer was just a small part of Patti's full life, but it changed her in several ways.

"Breast cancer made me love and respect every day that I live, even now, thirty-five years later. I care more for humanity and I'm much more compassionate."

Reflecting back on the more than three decades since being diagnosed with locally advanced breast cancer, Patti shares her insight as to why she has survived without hesitation.

"I believe that I survived breast cancer for all of these years because of my faith in the Lord and my joy in life. I questioned the Lord, 'What do you want of me? What can I do to praise you more for the life you've given me?' I follow His guidance and praise Him every day. I believe that I will be here on earth as long as the Lord has more work for me and then he will call me home."

Patti has enjoyed a healthy life after breast cancer until the need for a double knee replacement in early spring of 2014.

"I love my husband and the life that my Lord has blessed me with all of these years. I'm recovering from a double knee replacement but I feel like I'm forty. This is a great time in my life. Every day is more precious than the day before. I've come a long way in my seventy-nine years and I did it my way."

Looking to the future, Patti and Vince plan to continue enjoying their beautiful life together on the farm with their horses.

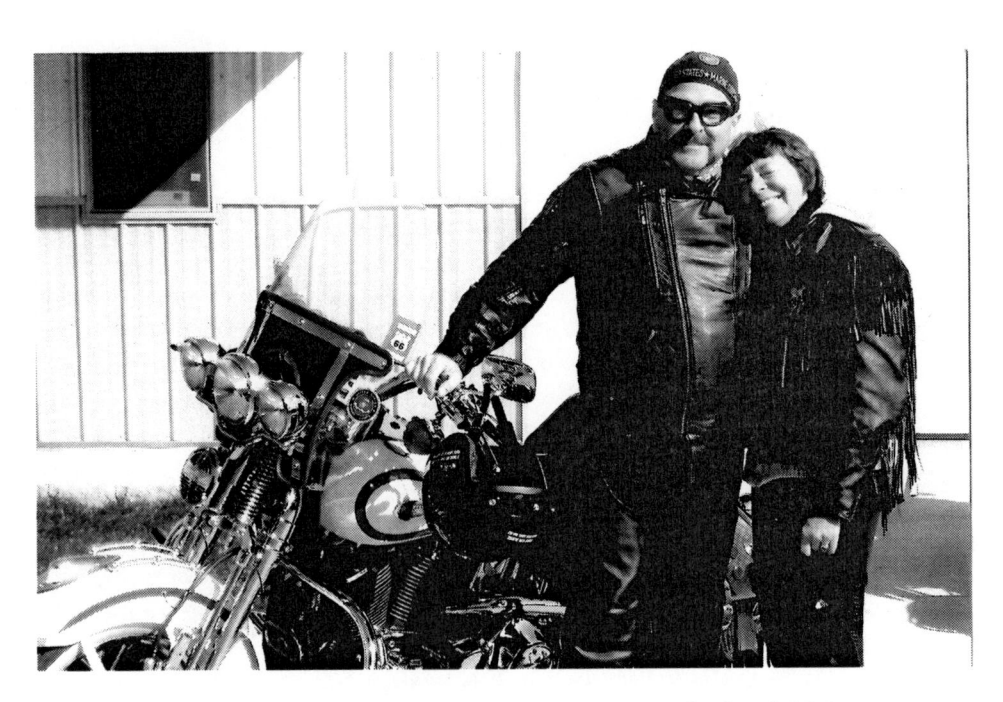

Jayne celebrating life after breast cancer with her husband, Hal!

CHAPTER 30 | Jayne Bailey

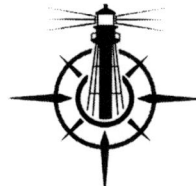

Celebrating Life Since She Was Diagnosed
in April 1990
Wauseon, OH

"God helped me through breast cancer treatment. There is always a little bit of fear of it coming back, but that had lessened with time. I know I'm past it."

Breast cancer was the last thing on Jayne's mind in the spring of 1990. Her work at a local hospital was fulfilling and her parental duties were evolving as her son and daughter entered their teen years. One steady constant in Jane's life was her husband, her lifelong love since the young age of twelve. She was forty-four years old when she discovered a lump in her breast. She didn't fit the profile for breast cancer. She was young, did not have a family history, and had been diligent with self-exams and mammograms. But she went to see her doctor immediately.

The results of the mammogram were concerning. A few days later, on her daughter's eighteenth birthday, she had a lumpectomy. Time stopped when she learned that she had breast cancer.

"I was so scared when I was diagnosed. In some ways, I think it was harder on my husband that it was me. I kept telling myself that I was going to get through it for my kids."

After analyzing the pathology report, her doctor decided that the tumor was just small enough to offset the need for chemotherapy. Radiation was the next step of treatment.

"We decided to visit Sanibel Island, Florida after my surgery and before radiation. Walking on the beach helped me feel closer to God. He never gives us a burden we can't handle."

After a trip filled with sand, sun, and prayer, Jayne was ready to start her radiation treatment. She never missed a day of work, but since the radiation made her weak, her family drove her to the hospital.

"My son drove me to my radiation treatments and we had a good time during those drives. It was a lot of fun spending that time with him. I stayed busy and never missed a day of work throughout my treatment."

Once treatment ended, Jayne healed physically, but she struggled with survivor's guilt. Fortunately, her work at the hospital allowed her to help others who were facing a breast cancer diagnosis. One of the highlights of Jayne's summer is gathering with other breast cancer survivors at the local fairgrounds in July. She offers hope and inspiration by sharing her story of survival with others.

"I'm more aware of how others feel when facing a difficult diagnosis. I can help them through the tough times by offering support and sharing my story."

Jayne has remained vigilant about self-exams and imaging since her diagnosis. She shares her insight into why she has survived breast cancer for twenty-five years and counting.

"I caught my breast cancer early and had knowledge of medicine because I had worked at the hospital and did a lot of research. I feel very fortunate that I've never had a recurrence. God helped me through breast cancer treatment and I've always been quick to call the doctor with any concerns. There is always a little bit of fear of it coming back, but that had lessened with time. I know I'm past it."

Breast cancer was Jayne's biggest challenge in life but the anniversary of her diagnosis no longer bothers her.

"My advice for anyone who is coping with breast cancer is to keep busy. Remember that every year is a good year."

Jayne recently celebrated her forty-seventh wedding anniversary with her husband. She lives close to both of her adult children and is very involved with their daily lives.

"We have a ball with our kids and grandkids. One of the highlights of my life was watching my granddaughter be born."

Now retired, Jayne plans to spend time spoiling her granddaughter and hopes to visit Hawaii someday in the future.

SECTION 4

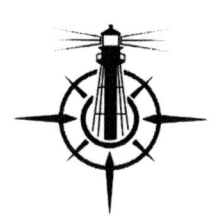

Defying the Odds

Statistics are invaluable in science and medicine. Treatment plans are developed based on the number of people who respond to a particular medication regimen at the time of the study. Proactive approaches are taken against the side effects experienced by the majority of patients. Prognosis is estimated based on statistics.

While numbers and graphs are necessary, they should never be used to eliminate hope. Even if the statistics are grim, doctors and patients should always consider that *someone* is that one percent or ten percent.

The women in this section were presented with the worst news an oncologist can deliver. Some were told to "get their affairs in order" and that they had mere months to live. Others were told they would never have children. But they defied the odds. They walked out of hospice, gave birth to children after chemotherapy, and met grandchildren decades after diagnosis.

Their stories are full of hope and inspiration that just might change the way you consider statistics.

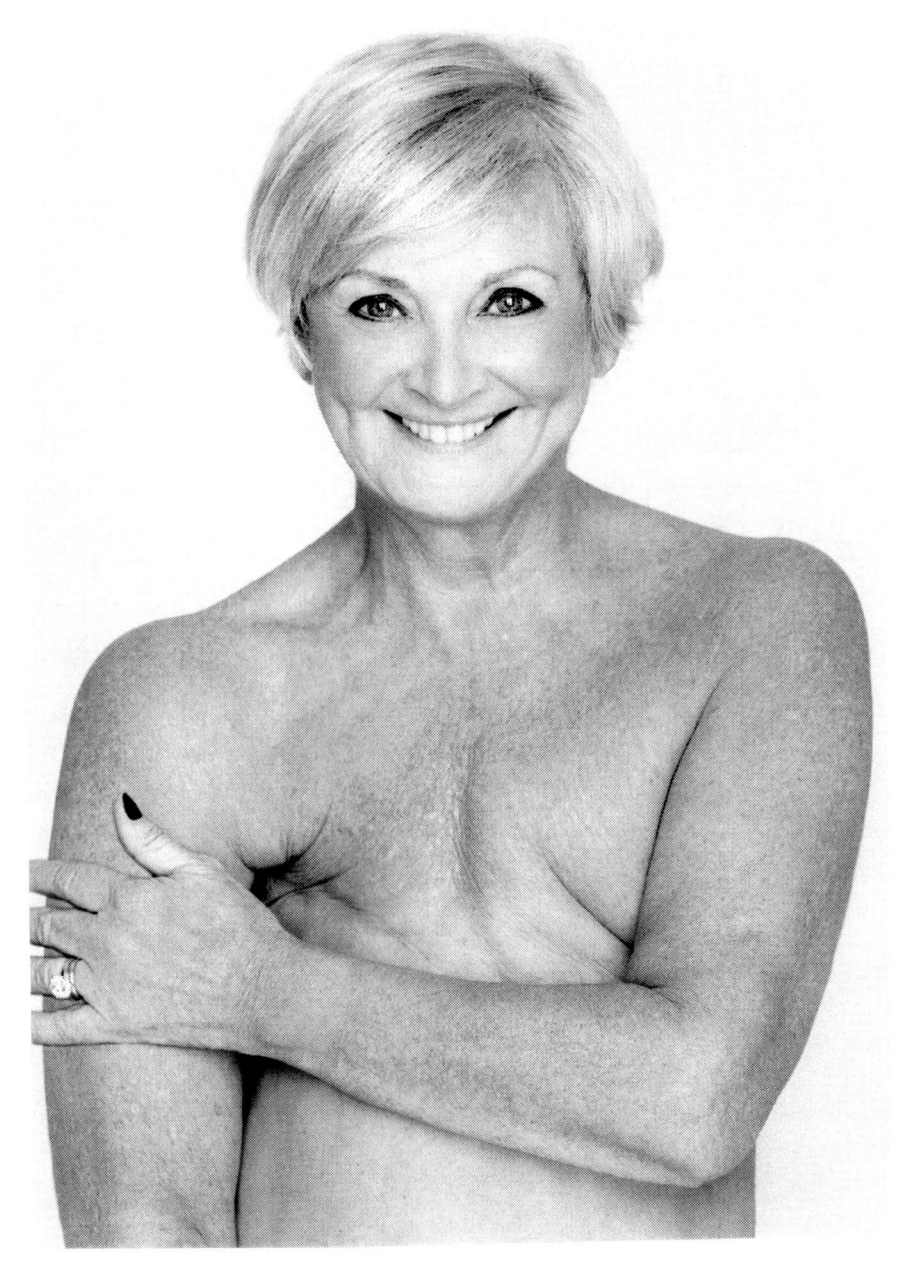

Dr. Jacqueline Kerr celebrating life after breast cancer with her inspirational photo shoot for a magazine two years after her second mastectomy.

CHAPTER 31 | Dr. Jacqueline Kerr

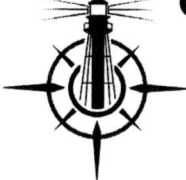

Celebrating Life Since She Was Diagnosed
in November 1992
New South Wales, Australia

"Even when I was in hospice, I never believed that I would die. The power of our thoughts is so important. I stayed positive and had a lot of support from my friends and family."

Dr. Jacqueline Kerr lived an extraordinary life in her early years. She grew up in both England and Australia and had traveled the world three times before her sixteenth birthday. She married an incredibly wealthy man and had five children at a very young age. The old adage that money does not buy happiness was certainly true in the case of Jacqueline's marriage. After enduring years of mental and physical abuse, she walked out of the relationship with nothing but a suitcase and her five young children.

After fourteen years as a single parent, Jacqueline took the opportunity to fulfill a lifelong dream and attend university.

"I'd always wanted to study but never had the opportunity. I enrolled in a social science program and being interested in family law I chose that for my honors. This area of study continued on to my PhD and I decided I could be of more help to women who were in abusive marriages. There weren't any anti-violence laws in Australia and I wanted to change that to protect other women."

As is often the case, Jacqueline's hard work and determination paid off. After Jacqueline completed her Bachelor of Social Science with honors, she went to Oxford and studied English Literature, followed by a postgraduate degree in applied psychology and a PhD in Jurisprudence. She enjoyed her role as an Associate Lecturer at the University of New South Wales.

"In March 1992 I was exactly where I'd always wanted to be. My children were independent and I was busy researching for my honors and enjoying my life. When I felt a lump in my breast and the doctor said it was nothing to worry about, I was not overly concerned."

The lump continued to grow in the months that followed. As she was busily preparing to give her dissertation, Jacqueline went back to see her doctor. She was sent for a mammogram during which the radiographer recommended an ultrasound. Her doctor disagreed, telling her that an ultrasound was unnecessary. Somewhere deep inside, Jacqueline's instincts told her to get a second opinion. She followed through with an ultrasound and shared the results with a new doctor.

On the very day that Jacqueline was scheduled to give her dissertation, she received an urgent call from her new doctor, insisting that she go to the hospital immediately. Many years of hard work had culminated into that day, so she made the decision to move forward with her dissertation.

"When I was admitted to the hospital the next day I was met by an oncologist who had studied the ultrasound. He asked me to sign a consent form in case he had to perform a mastectomy. It was only when he asked me who to call after the operation that I became concerned. I thought I was only there for a biopsy."

Still groggy from the anesthesia, Jacqueline's doctors shared the grim discovery they had made in the operating room.

"The doctor's words weren't making sense to me. The cancer has spread. You are too far gone, Jacqueline. We can't help you."

Recognizing the need for a more skilled surgeon, the doctors hadn't even attempted to remove the cancer. They had simply closed up the incision and arranged for Jacqueline to be transferred to a larger hospital. Her partner, John, had arranged for one of the top specialists in Australia to accept her case. Standard care at the time was a radical mastectomy but even this invasive surgery was not enough to remove all of the cancer. The surgical team had to remove bones, ribs, and lymph nodes in a surgery that lasted more than sixteen hours.

The pathology report indicated that the cancer had spread to more than half of Jacqueline's thirty-three lymph nodes. The doctors were straightforward about her prognosis. She would not survive. She might live two years based on their findings. Jacqueline shocked everyone with her reaction to this devastating news.

"I was certain I would beat it. It never occurred to me that I would not survive. I told them my life was all planned and I had too much to do. My best friend had been diagnosed with pancreatic cancer two weeks before my surgery so her situation was much more concerning than mine. I also had the support of my friends and family. My daughter had flown in from England, my sister from Perth, and my family from Queensland. Everyone came to see me and I was made to feel very special which was wonderful. I had more flowers than Cue Gardens and was really grateful."

Patients generally take time to recover from extensive surgery before starting chemotherapy but Jacqueline's case was different. Her team of doctors recommended a heavy dose of chemotherapy in addition to radiotherapy, a form of radiation.

"A mere four days after surgery, I was the first patient in Australia to receive radiotherapy and chemotherapy at the same time. My doctor told me that he hoped I had the strength to get through the treatment and warned me that I would lose my hair. In turn I told him I had always wanted to be a redhead anyway and now I could be any color I wanted. My family made every effort to make me comfortable and brought in my feather duvet and pillows, my Waterford crystal glasses, champagne and lots of glossy magazines. John filled the fridge with goodies and brought me fresh fruit and flowers every day. It was all very laid back and I had a ball with all of my visitors. I even snuck out to go shopping and to the opera in my nighties and dressing gowns. My parents flew in from Malta so that I could go home on the weekends while they cared for me. I was determined to remain positive and to stay as active as I could."

At first, the intense combination of treatment appeared to be working. Many months went by without incident until Jacqueline's entire immune system crashed resulting in a fever so high that she was placed into a special refrigerator unit for three days. She developed a severe case of shingles and her doctors discovered ten clots on her lungs. Less than a year after she was diagnosed, Jacqueline went to hospice.

In an unbelievable stroke of fate and coincidental timing, Jacqueline was placed into hospice with her friend who had been diagnosed with pancreatic cancer just weeks before Jacqueline's breast cancer diagnosis. They decided to make the most of their remaining days together.

Miraculously, Jacqueline's immune system recovered. Several months later, she walked out of hospice. Everyone was shocked, even her doctors. She was a living miracle. Jacqueline was determined to help others after leaving hospice but her biggest priority was her relationship with her partner John.

"A year after my surgery John and I traveled to America to visit my eldest daughter. We were married in Ensenada, Mexico, and we're still happily married to this day."

Breast cancer has not been a stranger in Jacqueline's life since her initial diagnosis. But after several surgeries, including a mastectomy in 2006, she has remained cancer free. She struggles with lymphedema and other side effects of treatment but enjoys every moment of every day. She is an advisory member of the National Breast Cancer Foundation and consultant for the Northern Rivers Health Commission and dedicates her time to helping others.

Recognizing the struggle with body image that often comes after breast cancer, Jacqueline was inspired to share her mastectomy scars in a very public way.

"I met a woman who had never shown her mastectomy scars to her husband. I showed her my scars and told her that she should be proud of her body because women are more than our breasts. My daughter was the editor-in-chief of a magazine at the time, so we decided to set up a photo shoot and publish the pictures in her magazine. I had a great experience with the photo shoot with an all-girl crew. The picture turned out well but most importantly, the article drew positive letters and saved lives."

Reflecting back over the last twenty-three years, Jacqueline shares her thoughts as to why she has survived breast cancer for more than two decades and counting.

"I never believed that I would die. The power of our thoughts is so important. I stayed positive and had a lot of support from my friends and family."

Jacqueline often uses the old Aborigine ritual of "point the bone" to explain the power of thought with the women that she counsels.

"Aborigines believe that they will die if a ritual expert points a bone at them as punishment for a crime. It is a sacred ceremony in which a large animal bone is simply pointed at the criminal. No one is touched by the bone or harmed in any way, but within weeks, the criminal grows weak and dies because he believes that he will die."

This story about the power of thought and Jacqueline's inspirational story have worked wonders for the women that she counsels, always pro bono.

"One woman I counseled had been told that she didn't have much time to live. Her markers kept going up and she was told by her oncologist to go home and accept she was going to die. I spent several months with her, helping change her outlook. After she went home from our first session, her mother rang and said 'thank you for sending my daughter back to me.' Unbelievably, over time, her markers started dropping and she is now in remission and her doctors cannot believe it."

Jacqueline's passion for counseling women with breast cancer has attracted attention from the medical field. She receives calls from doctors who have seen the effect that Jacqueline has on the patients.

"I once visited a ninety-seven-year-old Indian woman named Dorothy who was recovering from a mastectomy. She was upset because her surgeon had not offered her the option of reconstruction. I gave Dorothy six mastectomy bras and a small prosthesis. She was so excited that she stripped off her dress, put on the bra and was back in her dress in minutes. Dorothy immediately started clapping her hands and twirling around saying, 'Now I can get myself a boyfriend!' It was simply amazing. She is a wonderful woman and what a difference that prosthesis has made in her life."

Jacqueline is an active speaker, sharing her inspirational story of survival and is on a mission to help fund research for a cure for breast cancer. She also enjoys her role as legal guardian for World War II veterans.

"I tell others that given the choice, I would not change the fact that I had breast cancer. I don't want it again but it has taught me so much."

Jacqueline's children are all grown and live close to her. She enjoys spending time with her five wonderful grandchildren who are growing into amazing young adults. Looking to the future, she hopes to continue going on cruises with her husband, spoiling her grandchildren, and inspiring others with her amazing story of survival.

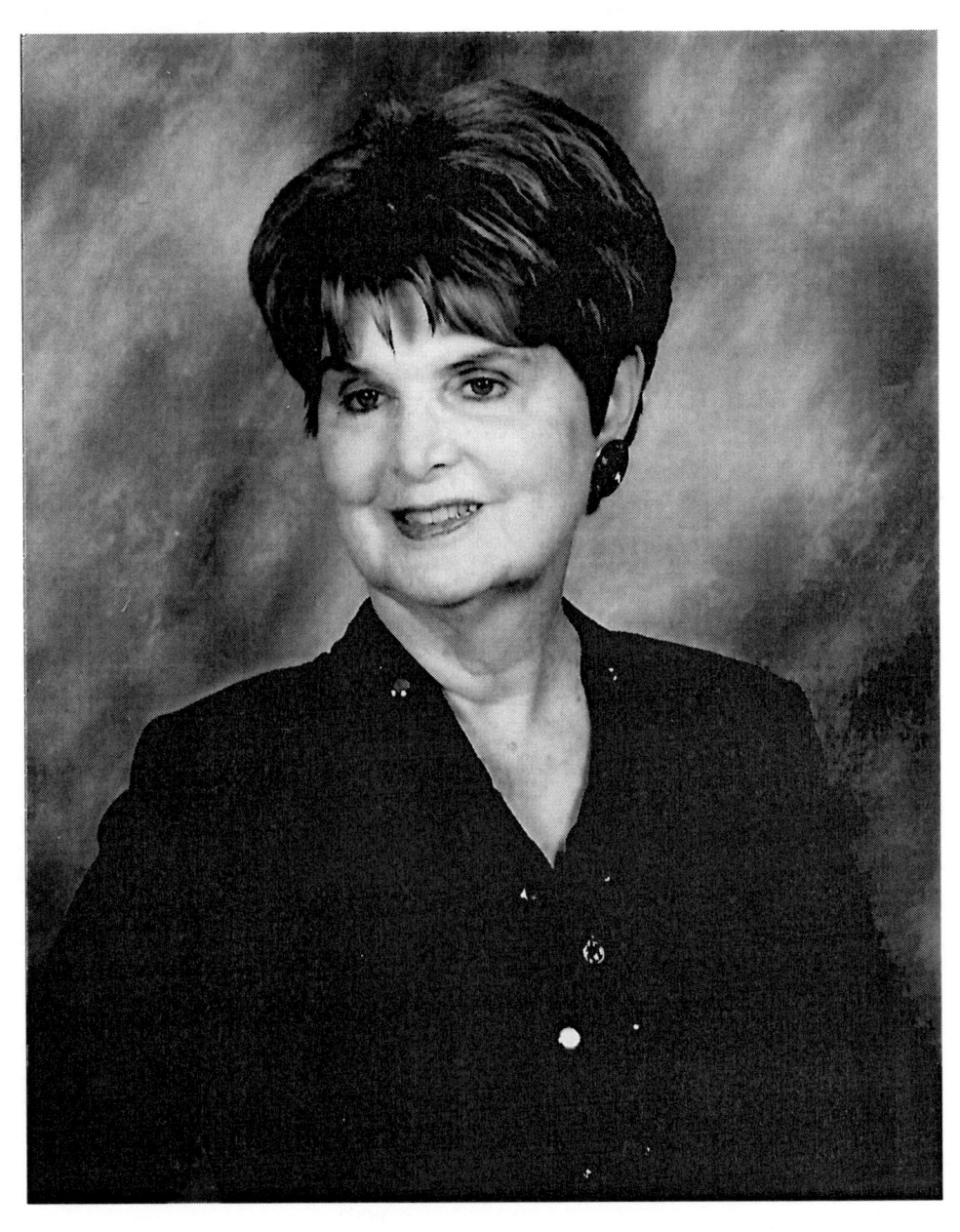

Marianne celebrating life after breast cancer just prior to her eightieth birthday

CHAPTER 32 | Marianne Werton

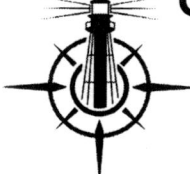

Celebrating Life Since She Was Diagnosed
in 1975 and 1977 (Stage IV)
Long Beach, CA

"Every happy experience was bittersweet, because I thought it would be my last one. One day, I decided to stop moping and start enjoying life."

Marianne traveled extensively as a young woman: Europe, Bermuda, St. Croix and Mexico were just a few of her many destinations over the years. But her greatest joy in life was her role as a mom to six children, ranging in grade from second to twelfth. Her busy life was interrupted when she found a lump in her breast.

A concerning event in any woman's life, Marianne's fear was intensified. She was still recovering from the loss of her mother to breast cancer. Things were different back then. Breast health was not discussed openly, so Marianne's mother had kept her lump a secret until it was too late. She died shortly after being diagnosed.

Marianne shared her fear and concern with her doctor, but he dismissed it, assuring her that she was fine. He insisted that she was too young for breast cancer and did not need a biopsy, sending her home with the plan to monitor any changes.

"I knew something was wrong in my gut. I was so aware of the lump, no matter what I was doing. I knew it was not right, but I followed the advice of my doctor. I wish I would have gone in for a second opinion."

She continued to visit her doctor every three months for a year. The ongoing appointments frustrated her doctor, which ultimately prompted him to do a needle aspiration. The goal was to alleviate Marianne's fears but the outcome was unexpected. The lump was not a cyst and needed to be biopsied.

"He told me that I needed to go to the hospital the next morning. One year of waiting and suddenly he felt it was urgent. I felt it was urgent from the moment I found the lump. Women should always trust their gut instinct."

A biopsy confirmed Marianne's worst fears. She had breast cancer. She stayed in the hospital for three days then had a radical mastectomy. She went home to recover but her journey was just beginning. Two months later, she had a recurrence on the scar line. One lump quickly multiplied into five lumps . . . all of which were surgically removed. Her cancer was very aggressive and the doctors hypothesized that surgery had made the tumor spread.

"The doctors were all arguing about my treatment plan right in front of us. They couldn't agree about whether we should do chemotherapy or radiation first. My husband, Jere, took my hand and we walked out of the doctor's office. We went home, determined to find the best doctors. We lived in Chicago at the time and our research led us to a doctor at a major hospital in Texas."

Her new doctor recommended eighteen months of chemotherapy, one treatment every twenty-eight days. A cocktail of three strong medications were administered on a gurney in her local doctor's office under the strict guidance of her specialist.

Radiation followed the chemotherapy regime followed by Tamoxifen. She also completed immunotherapy treatments with the goal of building up her immune system. Every three months, Marianne returned to Texas for follow-up testing with Jere beside her every step of the way.

It was a grueling journey, but she had many friends and neighbors who helped with meals and transportation to appointments. Her biggest goal was to keep everything as normal at home with her children as possible. Everyone breathed a sigh of relief when treatment ended. Unfortunately, Marianne's journey through breast cancer was still not complete.

"We were devastated when I found a new lump only three months after finishing chemotherapy. My specialist referred us to a different major hospital for a new regimen. We traveled for days to meet with new doctors, but they wanted us to sign a waiver that said if I died while in their treatment, they could keep my body for research. Jere refused to sign that waiver, so they refused to treat me. We went back home and started over. It was so frightening."

Back home, Marianne had surgery to remove the new lump. No one could have predicted the grim discovery that would be made on the operating table.

"The cancer had spread to my bones and I was now considered Stage IV. The surgeon removed my ribs until they had clean margins. Recovery was very difficult and the doctors recommended more chemotherapy. My husband and I discussed it and we refused further treatment. We decided to lean on prayer and faith, since nothing else seemed to be working."

The physical and emotional impact of treatment, ongoing recurrences and a new Stage IV diagnosis took their toll on Marianne.

"I lost my power to think and do for myself at some point. I was completely dependent on my husband to make all of the treatment decisions. I leaned so heavily on him. I would wake him up in the middle of the night and ask him to hold me. One night, it was very late and I was so overwhelmed. I asked him if he would just let me go the easy way. I was so tired and afraid. He said there was no easy way and that I wasn't going anywhere. He gave me the strength and support to get through that long night and to keep moving forward in the days that followed."

Marianne began to regain her strength as the months passed. She prayed constantly but the fear was always present.

"Every happy experience was bittersweet, because I thought it would be my last one. I spent every day thinking that I would die within a year. My biggest fear was leaving my children without a mother. I wanted to start interviewing caregivers to watch over the kids after I was gone but Jere said no way."

Months went by and Marianne healed physically but continued to struggle emotionally.

"I was living in such fear for so long. Then my neighbor died suddenly from a heart attack and it changed me. I decided to stop moping and start living and enjoying life each day."

As the months turned into years, Marianne's children grew older and began lives of their own. It took time, but she came to realize that breast cancer had changed her as a person.

"Breast cancer deepened my faith in God and gave me a new level of appreciation for my husband. I learned to empathize with other people and to appreciate every day. Later in life, I learned that there are worse things than breast cancer. Seeing my adult children struggle and my own daughter diagnosed with breast cancer has been much more difficult than my own journey."

Four decades have passed since Marianne was first diagnosed with breast cancer and later re-diagnosed with metastasis. She shares her insight about why she believes she has survived for so long after such a harrowing journey.

"I believe that I am still here today because I found good doctors and had faith. I prayed constantly for my doctors and that the treatment would work. I had faith that I would make it through but when my faith wavered, I leaned on my husband. Once treatment ended, we moved to a new state for a fresh start in life which helped me live a normal life."

Marianne recently celebrated her eightieth birthday with her daughters and their families. She travels the country to visit her children and grandchildren and continues to appreciate every day. As she contemplates her life and looks to the future, Marianne shares the highlight of her life and one last item on her bucket list.

"My biggest joy in life has been raising my six children and ten grandchildren. There was a time that I was afraid I wouldn't be here to see my kids reach adulthood and now they are all living their own lives with their own families. I've done everything in life that I've ever wanted to do but I have one last thing on my bucket list. I would like to have all of my family together one last time. It's difficult to find a time when all six children and all of the grandchildren can come together but that's my hope for the future."

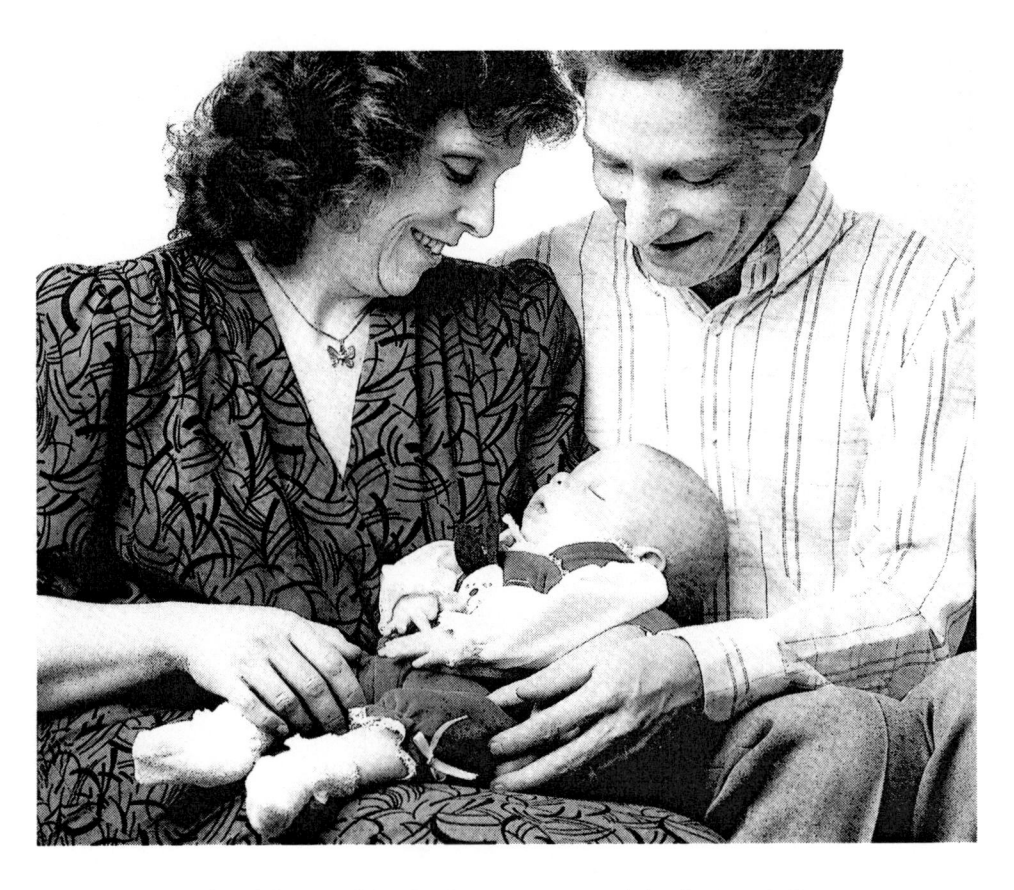

Linda celebrating life after breast cancer with her husband, Steve, and their beautiful baby girl, Amanda.

CHAPTER 33 | Linda Radick

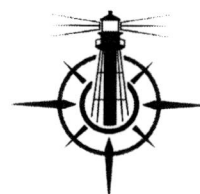

Celebrating Life Since She Was Diagnosed
in 1982 and 1986
St. Louis, MO

"We focused on the positive and welcomed my daughter into the world. Two years later, we welcomed my son. As far as my plastic surgeon knew, I was only the third person in the world to have children after a TRAM flap surgery."

Life on the road was exhilarating for Linda. She was touring the country with her band, Ron Furr's "A Touch of Elvis," without a care in the world. One evening, she was preparing to play keyboard and sing back-up for a show in Jacksonville, Florida. Something unexpected caught her attention in the mirror: a lump in her breast, the size of an egg, had appeared out of nowhere.

"Breast cancer did not run in my family and I was young, but I knew it was breast cancer. As they say, the show must go on, so I performed in a fog that night."

Far away from home, Linda talked to her band members and the stage manager, who referred her to a local doctor. The next twenty-four hours were a blur. The local doctor tried unsuccessfully to aspirate the lump and referred her to a surgeon. After a quick exam, surgery was scheduled for the next morning. The band was in shock but went on to perform for their loyal audience that evening.

"I refused to let them do a mastectomy. I was young, unmarried and felt my life would be over if I got a mastectomy. During surgery, the doctor came out to ask my fellow band members for permission to do a mastectomy. They said no, which made the doctor so mad. He refused to come tell me it was cancer until later that night."

Linda was diagnosed with a very rare type of breast cancer: clear-cell carcinoma. She took a break from the band and moved back to St. Louis to recover under the watchful eye of her parents. A local surgeon shared upsetting news after a lymph node dissection. The cancer had spread to Linda's lymph nodes and the outlook was grim.

"The doctor told me that he wasn't going to make me have a mastectomy because he didn't think anything would save me. Later, a nun came in and told me that I should accept God's plan and not fight. My mother was crying and I was devastated. I had always wanted a family and children and it was too late. For six weeks, I thought I was a dead woman."

Hope came in the form of an upbeat oncologist who became so involved with her case that he later attended her wedding. His plan of attack was twenty months of very difficult chemotherapy.

"Times were different back then. I was so very sick with every chemo treatment. Eventually, my veins gave out so they put in a Hickman catheter. I was so lonely and there was very little cancer support at that time. All I could think about was getting back together with my band. They held my spot and after a year and a half, I was back on the road with them."

Life with the band was fun, but something inside Linda had changed. She had started dating fellow band member/long-time friend, Steve, during treatment and knew that she wanted to settle down and get married in the future. At the age of thirty-five, Linda quit the band and got a day job. She was delighted when Steve left the band to start a new life with her. They both played in bands on the weekends and were enjoying life when breast cancer struck again.

"The lump that I thought was scar tissue turned out to be a recurrence. This time, I was blessed to be in a relationship with a man who didn't care about anything other than me surviving, so I had a mastectomy."

Watching a loved one cope with cancer can be emotionally challenging for anyone. Steve had watched his former band member/long-time friend/now girlfriend fight breast cancer twice. This time, he realized just how much she meant to him and he proposed.

"Life was good. We were planning our future together and we both wanted to become parents. But my oncologist had warned me that pregnancy following the strong chemotherapy drugs was unlikely. He also asked me if I really wanted to take the chance that I would have a child who would have to grow up without a mother."

Linda moved forward with the next phase in her breast cancer journey. She underwent TRAM flap surgery, which involves a long incision across the middle of the abdomen to move abdominal muscle and tissue up to the chest. It was an extensive surgery but she was pleased with the results.

"After recovering from TRAM flap surgery, an all-consuming fatigue came over me. I could barely keep my eyes open at work and I was exhausted all of the time. I just knew the cancer was back and I was so afraid."

A co-worker suggested a pregnancy test, but Linda assured her that wasn't necessary. Her oncologist's words echoed throughout her brain, telling her she would never become a parent. But statistics do not always predict the future. Linda's worst fear of recurrence turned into the greatest joy of her life the day she discovered that she was indeed pregnant!

"Everyone was excited about the pregnancy except some of my relatives in the medical field. They were terrified that the cancer would come back because of the hormones. We focused on the positive and welcomed my daughter into the world. Two years later, we welcomed my son. As far as my plastic surgeon knew, I was only the third person in the world to have children after a TRAM flap surgery. I was forty years old with a newborn and a toddler."

Linda dealt with the normal struggles after breast cancer, such as being fearful with every new ache or pain. There were times when she worried about surviving long enough to raise her children, especially after a scare when the kids were six and eight. She feels blessed that she remained cancer free.

Many new chapters in life have come and gone for Linda, including several day jobs, occasionally playing with bands on the weekends, work as a music minister, and most recently, her job as a freelance pianist and piano instructor. She volunteers at her local cancer center once per week, where she fills the otherwise solemn lobby with beautiful music. She brings a smile to everyone's face with her talent and passion for music and for life.

"I was delighted to turn forty, then fifty and sixty. I have so much gratitude with each birthday. My husband and I have enjoyed raising our children who are now adults in their mid-twenties. It's been a good run!"

Reflecting over her life since her first diagnosis, Linda shares her insight as to why she has survived breast cancer for more than three decades.

"I believe we are all where we are supposed to be. My life has God's thumbprint all over it and breast cancer helped me become more spiritual. I also believe that my inner strength and the support of friends and family helped me through. I was amazed at what I could endure in order to get well again. It was all worth it."

Looking to the future, spending time with her family is at the top of Linda's list. She plans to continue sharing her talent of piano performances and volunteering at her local cancer center. A trip to Europe with her husband is another dream for the future but it may not compare to her favorite adventure in life to date.

"We went on an Alaskan cruise and it was phenomenal! It truly was the best trip ever!"

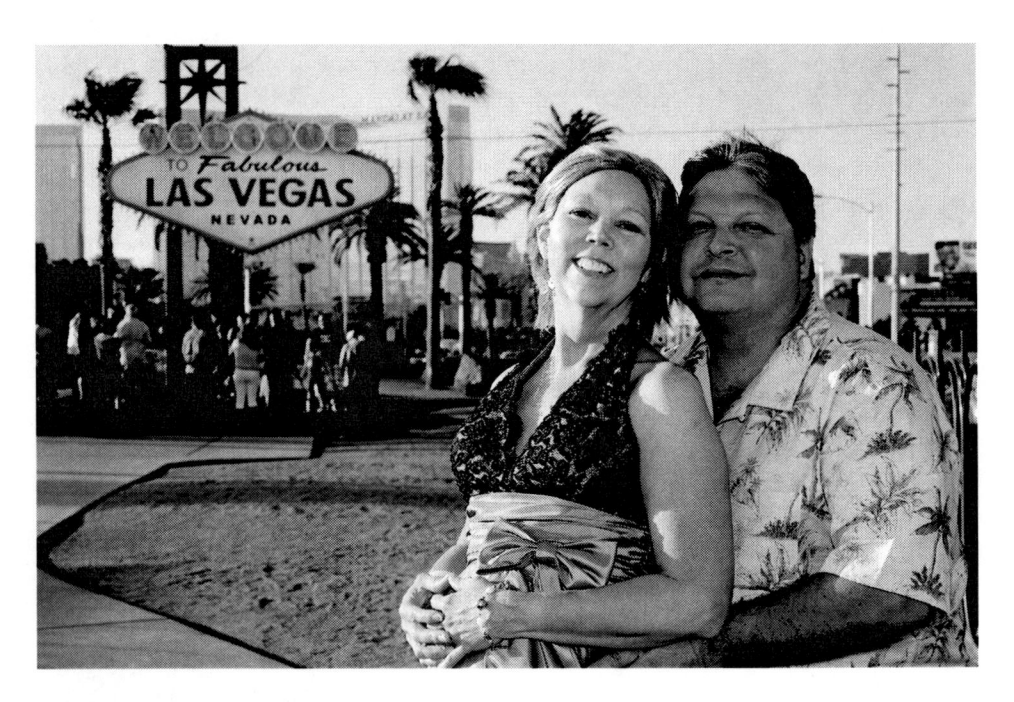

Debbie celebrating life after breast cancer with her husband, just after renewing their wedding vows in Las Vegas for their twenty-year anniversary!

CHAPTER 34 | Debbie Davis

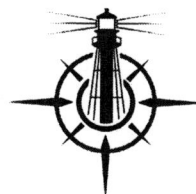

Celebrating Life Since She Was Diagnosed
in 1993, 1996, and 2000 (Stage IV)
St. Louis, MO

"Everyone is good at something. I never had a niche until I was diagnosed. I'm good at being a breast cancer survivor."

A newlywed, Debbie was loving life with her new husband. Looking forward to starting a family, she wasn't overly concerned when she discovered a lump under her arm. A visit to her obstetrician resulted in a mammogram and then a biopsy. One week later, Debbie received the news that would change her life . . . she had breast cancer.

After discussing the options with her doctor, she had a lumpectomy and a lymph node dissection. The pathology report indicated that the cancer has spread to three of twenty-one lymph nodes. Chemotherapy wasn't easy, but Debbie continued to work out and stay healthy.

"I didn't want looks of pity from strangers, so I always wore my wig, even when I worked out. After I finished a month of radiation, I went on with my life. My husband's grandmother had survived breast cancer for forty years so I had a good role model."

Two years after completing chemotherapy and radiation, Debbie received the shock of a lifetime.

"I was pregnant! We couldn't believe it. The doctors had told us we probably wouldn't be able to have children. We were so lucky to have my son and we love him so much."

Debbie had a recurrence three years after her first diagnosis so she opted for a mastectomy. She healed physically and emotionally and put her energy into raising her miracle baby. Her son was five when she went in for a routine scan in 2000. No one was prepared for the results of that scan. Her breast cancer had metastasized to her skull. Over the next few years, the cancer spread to her other breast, bones, chest wall, and liver.

"It was very difficult every time the cancer came back. Multiple surgeries and hormone therapy including clinical trials have worked for varying amounts of time. Once I tried all of the hormone therapy, my doctor recommended traditional chemotherapy and radiation again. I have never been afraid to try clinical trials and some have surprised us at how well they have worked. I have faith that there will always be something new for me to try when I need it."

Debbie learned that there has been a shift in thinking among oncologists about clinical trials. Until recently, doctors have treated Stage IV breast cancer with the standard treatment options first, resorting to clinical trials if the tumors do not respond. Now, doctors will often begin with a clinical trial, resorting to traditional options if needed. New clinical trials are always on the horizon, offering hope to women facing metastasis.

"I get a lot of my positive attitude and hope from knowing that there are always more upcoming clinical trials. They have the potential to help me and so many others and help us inch closer to a cure."

Debbie takes an active role in her treatment, researching side effects and benefits of each of her treatment options.

"I have a lot of trust and faith in my doctor. I know he puts a great deal of thought into which clinical trials are right for me. I research each clinical trial myself and have never been afraid to start one."

Stage IV breast cancer is considered by many oncologists to be a chronic disease, meaning that it will never be cured but can often be treated. Debbie's doctor has a different goal in mind.

"My oncologist specializes in patients whose breast cancer has metastasized. His goal is to cure Stage IV breast cancer. He's an amazing doctor. I go to my cancer center every three weeks for treatment. It has just become a part of my life. I keep a spreadsheet of all of the treatments that I've received as well as the results."

The assumption by many is that people with Stage IV breast cancer will receive chemotherapy for the rest of their lives. This has not been the case for Debbie. Her doctor initially formulated a treatment plan that involved traditional hormonal therapies, trying different ones including a clinical trial with various degrees of success. This treatment approach lasted for seven years. She has participated in several chemotherapy and radiation clinical trials over the last six years, enjoying long stretches without progression, some more than a year.

"I recently had radioembolization to treat the tumors in my liver. This involves putting tiny radioactive beads into my liver tumor through my hepatic artery. Recently, I learned that the tumor shank from 6 cm x 4 cm to 8 mm x 8 mm. It was great news!"

Reflecting back on her life and experiences with breast cancer, Debbie is grateful for the support she has received from family and friends. She refuses to allow her mind to go down the dangerous road of "what if," instead surrounding herself with positive people.

"My husband reminds me constantly that I'll be fine. I seek out people who are positive and never let my mind go anywhere but positive. It took me a long time to Google my type of breast cancer as I don't care about statistics."

Breast cancer has brought many changes into Debbie's life, including her job. She helps maintain a website designed to keep everyone informed about the very latest medical research related to many types of diseases, including breast cancer. She scours the Internet for newly released articles about breast cancer, reviews them, and then posts them to the website.

"Breast cancer has changed my life in every possible way. I wouldn't be the person I am today if I hadn't been diagnosed. My personality has changed completely. I used to be shy but now I get in front of groups to talk about my journey."

Debbie doesn't hesitate when asked why she believes she has survived twenty-three years since her initial breast cancer diagnosis and fifteen years since her Stage IV diagnosis.

"Breast cancer has given me a purpose in life. I have never let my mind go anywhere but the positive. I am a twenty-three-year breast cancer survivor . . . it's who I am. I feel great right now and the cancer does not slow down my lifestyle at all, in fact it actually enhances it. I work out, stay busy with work, and I've been very involved with my son. I believe I will beat this disease. Everyone is good at something. I never had a niche until I was diagnosed. I am good at being a breast cancer survivor."

Debbie's son, who was born three years after her initial diagnosis, is all grown up now. She is helping him with college deadlines and the normal everyday things that teenagers experience. She feels fortunate that she has watched him grow into an amazing young man.

"I have enjoyed being very involved with my son's school and his childhood. He is a typical teenager. I always have fun with him and with life in general. Not because life will end but because that's who I am. I plan to keep having fun with my family and friends for many years."

Looking ahead, Debbie looks forward to continuing with her work.

"The future is so bright in terms of research, especially with personalized medicine. I believe we are so close to a cure for breast cancer which will be a dream come true. On a personal level, I have the option of reconstruction. Who knows, maybe I will get new boobs for my sixtieth birthday!"

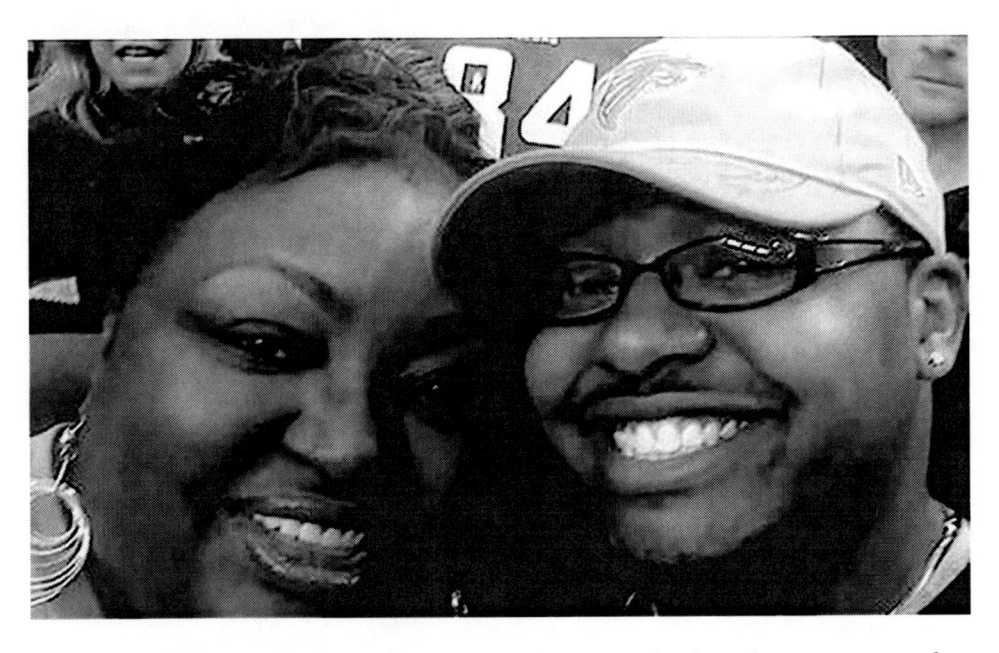

Beverly celebrating life after breast cancer with her son, Roland, as she was receiving the Dazzle of Hope Award for her volunteer work in 2012.

CHAPTER 35
Beverly Hunter Anderson

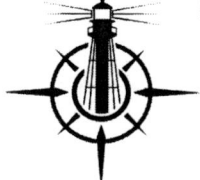

Celebrating Life Since She Was Diagnosed
in April 1983
Stone Mountain, GA

"I thought I was the only black woman with breast cancer. I was only twenty-six years old. It helped to know that someone else had survived it for a long time."

Motherhood is a true blessing but can often be overwhelming. Beverly loved her nine-month-old little girl, but she was delighted to have a day to herself to enjoy the finer things in life, like a long, uninterrupted shower.

"I was singing in the shower, so happy to have the day to myself. I had learned to do self-breast exams in high school and I had time to do one that morning. That's when I found something in my breast. I thought it was a mosquito bite, so I rinsed off and looked for a red mark, but there wasn't anything visible. I jumped out of the shower, dried off and got some baby powder so my skin would be smooth. I had baby powder all over that bathroom and I felt the lump again. I remember thinking, 'I have cancer. I'm going to die.' My boyfriend came home and he could feel the lump too. I was in a panic."

Beverly did not want to alert her family but she was terrified. She found reasons to avoid making an appointment until her boyfriend threatened to tell her mom. She decided to see a doctor at the health clinic where she was working as a pharmacy technician.

"I didn't even know what a mammogram was . . . I was only twenty-six years old. I had to go to the hospital for a mammogram, sonogram, and some other test. One week later, I was sitting in the back room of the clinic, waiting for my results. I waited so long that I finally came out and everyone was gone except me and one nurse. I thought they had forgotten about me but the doctor was on his way. He told me that it was probably nothing but I got so upset that he agreed to do a biopsy, just to reassure me that I was fine."

Beverly finally shared her fears with her family, friends, and coworkers, which started a revolving door of visitors. Their prayers and support offered comfort while waiting for the results of the biopsy. She went in to have her incision checked one week after the biopsy, feeling confident that she was too young for breast cancer.

"I was joking and flirting with my handsome doctor while he checked my incision. We were finishing up when I said, 'By the way, what were the results of my biopsy?' He hadn't even checked them but he told me they were probably fine. He opened my chart and started rubbing his eyes. I could see tears forming. He told me he would be back in a minute and I remember looking out his office window. He came back with the medical team . . . six young white guys. They were all crying. My doctor couldn't speak because he was so choked up. One of the other guys told me it was malignant and they would need to remove my breast. They wanted to schedule my appointment but I kept telling them I couldn't leave my baby. Then I couldn't hear what they were saying anymore. All I heard was 'wamp, wamp, wamp' . . . just like Charlie Brown's teacher. I was just staring out the window when I heard the word, 'okay' and a nurse took my arm to walk me out of the office."

Recognizing the need for support, the nurse offered to call Beverly's mom, who also worked in the clinic. She declined the offer and walked back to the pharmacy where she worked. She was in shock but began to type a letter to her boss, requesting time off for surgery.

"My coworker walked in all happy, assuming I had received good news. She asked me if I was okay because I was so quiet, which is not like me at all. I started crying and opened my mouth to tell her my news. I could hear someone screaming and I kept thinking that person needed to stop screaming. It was so loud and kept going on and on. Then I realized . . . I was the one screaming. I was hysterical. They gave me a valium and within thirty minutes, I was floating on a cloud. I looked around and my mama was there with my friends and coworkers. They were all crying but I had no idea why."

Beverly's mom took her home and then shared a secret with her. A good family friend was a breast cancer survivor. Three decades ago, people didn't talk about breast cancer, especially within the African American community.

"I thought I was the only black woman with breast cancer. It helped to know that someone else had survived it for a long time. It was not an easy weekend but everyone was visiting me and praying. I tried to go back to work that week but everyone kept crying. I finally told my boss that I couldn't take care of everyone else and myself so I stayed home until the day of my surgery. It just happened to be Mother's Day that weekend, my first one as a mom but it was not a good one because of the fear."

Beverly had a unilateral mastectomy and lymph node dissection one day after Mother's Day. The support from friends and family throughout her two-week stay was beyond anyone's expectation.

"I had a huge welcome back from the recovery room. I had no idea that so many people could fit into one hospital room. My friends delivered homemade meals to my hospital room every day. They surprised me with a metal money tree full of ten- and twenty-dollar bills."

The pathology report indicated that the cancer was in at least one, possibly two lymph nodes. The doctors decided she was too young for radiation, but she would need six months of chemotherapy.

"At first, I had a pity party for myself but then a close friend who is a nurse took charge. She told me I was getting out of bed. She took out my IV and helped me walk down the hall. After that, I would walk the hospital floors at night, visiting the babies and thinking about everything."

After two weeks in the hospital, Beverly went home. She had lots of support to care for her baby and many unexpected sources of help.

"A rep from a short-term disability company had visited me at work just before I was diagnosed. I had made one payment on the policy but they paid for the work that I missed. I had free diapers for a year and free formula for three months. I never knew I had so many friends."

Four weeks after surgery, Beverly started a six-month regimen of chemotherapy. She had a combination of three drugs and the side effects were challenging. She lived alone and needed constant help to care for her daughter.

"I had low points but I just kept going for my daughter. My baby would stay with my mom because I was too sick to take care of her. I had a friend who started coming to check on me every day. He would sleep on the couch so I wouldn't be alone at night. He was the only person who ever saw me cry. We're still friends to this day."

Once chemotherapy was complete, Beverly went back to work. As the years passed, everything moved in a positive direction. Less than four years after being diagnosed, Beverly got married. She was delighted to learn that she was pregnant again, but the surge of hormones with pregnancy was concerning for her doctor. Everyone was relieved when she delivered a healthy baby girl.

"I had been on maternity leave for six months and felt great. Suddenly, I was tired and didn't feel good. I was scared that the cancer was back so I had a friend who was a physician's assistant do an exam. It turns out, I was pregnant. Again. My doctor had a fit and encouraged me to have an abortion. I told him, 'My mamma says that God takes care of children, women, and fools. I'm having this baby.' I had some complications but my son was born healthy. I had my tubes tied during my c-section so I wouldn't have any more children."

Beverly continued on with life as a busy mom of three children. She had reconstruction and a breast reduction on the other side. She later had problems with chronic fatigue and other mysterious symptoms. The doctors discovered that her implant had ruptured, so she had it removed and did not opt for any further reconstruction.

"I've had one breast most of my life so it was not a big deal. I have a nice prosthesis but usually don't wear it around the house. My sexuality is not about my breast. I know women sometimes delay treatment because they are afraid to lose a breast but you should never make a decision about your health based on the fear of your husband leaving you. If that happens, God will send someone to love you."

Breast cancer changed Beverly's life in many ways. She has always been in high demand to offer support to other young women. She volunteered with Bosom Buddies and changed her career focus to outreach. She worked as a patient navigator for many years which led to appearances on radio talk shows. At one point, she represented the hospital as a young breast cancer survivor.

"I was one of the young women with breast cancer who went on to have children. I inspired other women to have their own families after their treatment. I got a lot out of it throughout the years. I never want to see anyone join the sorority of breast cancer sisters but once you are in, you are in it forever. You'll never be alone."

One of the highlights of Beverly's journey through breast cancer has been her participation in a nationally recognized all-breast cancer survivor choir.

"I cannot sing but I make a joyful sound onto the Lord. We have traveled all over the country and have been on television. It's just awesome to be a part of Shades of Pink. Once you are in the choir, you are family."

Reflecting back on her journey through breast cancer, Beverly shares her insight as to why she has survived breast cancer for more than three decades and counting.

"I don't have a secret to longevity. I had youth on my side and I believe that God has a reason for keeping me here. He wasn't finished using me and had work for me to do. Maybe His plan was for me to help others so I try to give back as much as possible. I have been there for lots of women throughout the years. I know that I'll see His plan when it's time. I also think that it helped that I never asked 'why me?' I know you have to be positive to heal because healing is 50% attitude."

With breast cancer long in her past, Beverly no longer dwells on the possibility of recurrence. She has yearly mammograms and moves on with her goal of helping other women. Her children are all grown up and leading productive lives of their own. Her favorite role in life came about with the birth of her grandson.

"One of the greatest joys in my life has been this grandbaby. I never thought I would see my own grandchildren. I love being 'nana' to this little boy. He is my heart. We have so much fun together."

Beverly enjoys going on annual Breast Cancer Thriver's Cruises with hundreds of breast cancer survivors and their caregivers. She loves visiting new places, spending time with old friends, and meeting new women. Back at home, she enjoys event planning for families and friends. Her experience with breast cancer has given her an inner strength that has helped her cope with the many challenges that she has been faced with throughout her life.

"When things happen to me, I remember that I survived breast cancer so I can survive anything. I've been knocked down at times but I keep smiling and keep on going."

Looking to the future, Beverly is optimistic about life. She is considering going back to school to get a Master's Degree in Public Health and wants to start her own nonprofit organization that will help women and children. She doesn't plan to slow down anytime in the near future.

"I've been incredibly blessed in my life. I feel good about my future. I'm almost sixty years old and plan to live another sixty years. My number-one goal is to spoil my grandson."

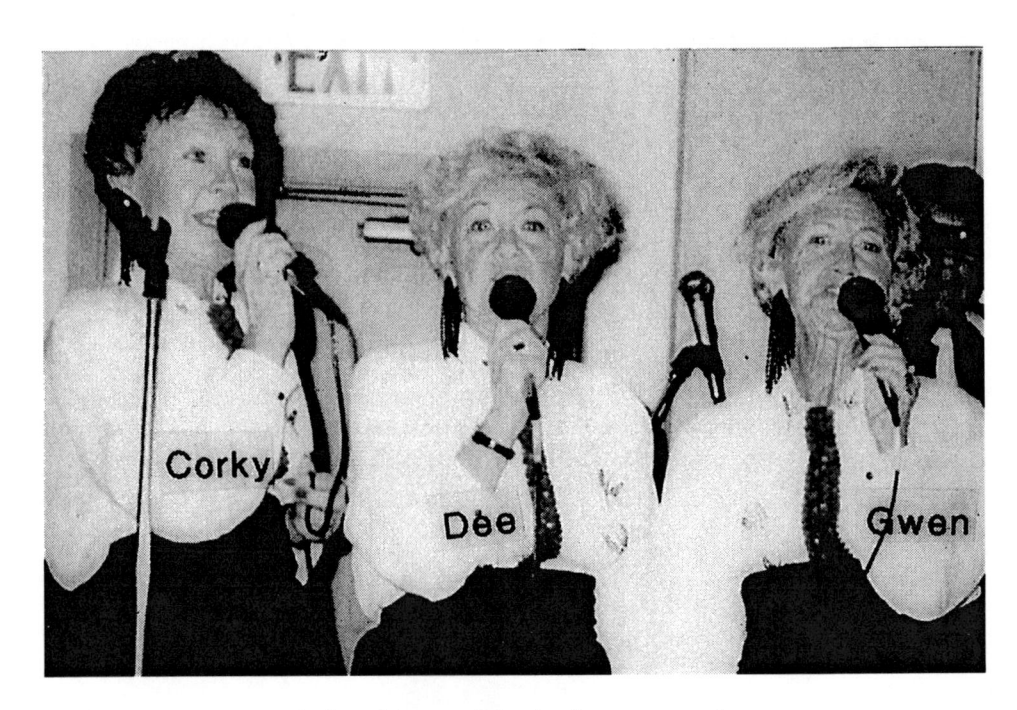

Corky celebrating life after breast cancer by singing in the band with her sisters!

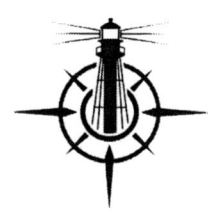

CHAPTER 36 | Corky Ellis

Celebrating Life Since She Was Diagnosed in
1967 and 1970 (Stage IV)
Huntington Beach, California

"It was very scary knowing that the cancer had spread to other parts of my body. I realize now that I was one of the lucky ones."

Corky's life has been full of adventure. A music lover since the moment she was born, she started a band with her sisters as a young teen. Performing for friends and family was great fun so they expanded their repertoire to nursing homes. Their musical talent attracted attention locally, leading them to play in nightclubs. They produced several CDs which landed them on the radio.

"I had the time of my life singing with my sisters so many years ago! I listen to my CDs and smile at the many fun memories."

She was a busy wife, mom, and musician when she found a lump at the age of forty. She wasn't overly concerned but made time to see the doctor.

"I didn't think it was cancer, so I wasn't worried. I went to see the doctor and was shocked to learn it was cancer."

The standard treatment at the time was a radical mastectomy. The surgery was invasive but successful. As she began to heal physically, she struggled with weakness on her right side. The emotional impact of surgery was more difficult than the physical side effects.

"I was so very sad when I woke up from surgery. I was depressed over having lost my boob. I felt very sorry for myself for several months but eventually life goes on."

The treatment options were very limited nearly five decades ago, so Corky was not offered further treatment or reconstruction. Corky leaned on her husband and family for support but the diagnosis was isolating at the time.

"Things were different all those years ago. People didn't really talk about it so I didn't discuss my experience with anyone other than my family."

Three years later, breast cancer paid another visit. This time it was metastatic, having spread to other parts of her body. Corky underwent additional surgery, including removing her kidney in an effort to eradicate the disease.

"It was very scary knowing that the cancer had spread to other parts of my body. I realize now that I was one of the lucky ones. I had good doctors who helped me get through it. I'm just thankful that it all went well and the cancer never came back after that."

Always the optimist, Corky found positives through her experience with breast cancer.

"I found out what a wonderful husband and family that I had because of my diagnosis. I learned to appreciate them more every day."

Corky has enjoyed a full life after surviving breast cancer twice. She raised her children, spoiled her grandchildren, and now enjoys her great-grandchildren. Looking back, Corky shares her insight as to why she has survived for nearly five decades.

"I did everything my doctor told me to do and I had faith that I would get through it. Attitude is so important and a sense of humor helps too."

Corky practices an attitude of gratitude daily.

"I am grateful that I have a wonderful family. I enjoy waking up every morning and enjoy a new day. I feel very fortunate that I can look back on a full life and smile at the many memories that I have created with my friends and family."

Breast cancer recently entered Corky's life in a different way. Her daughter was diagnosed and went through chemotherapy.

"I wish I could have helped my daughter more with her chemotherapy. When I see what she went through, my own journey was so much easier. But I have faith that she will come out stronger on the other side."

Looking to the future, Corky has a short bucket list.

"I've done everything that I've ever wanted to do in my life. At this point, I would love to meet more great-grandchildren and continue to enjoy my wonderful family."

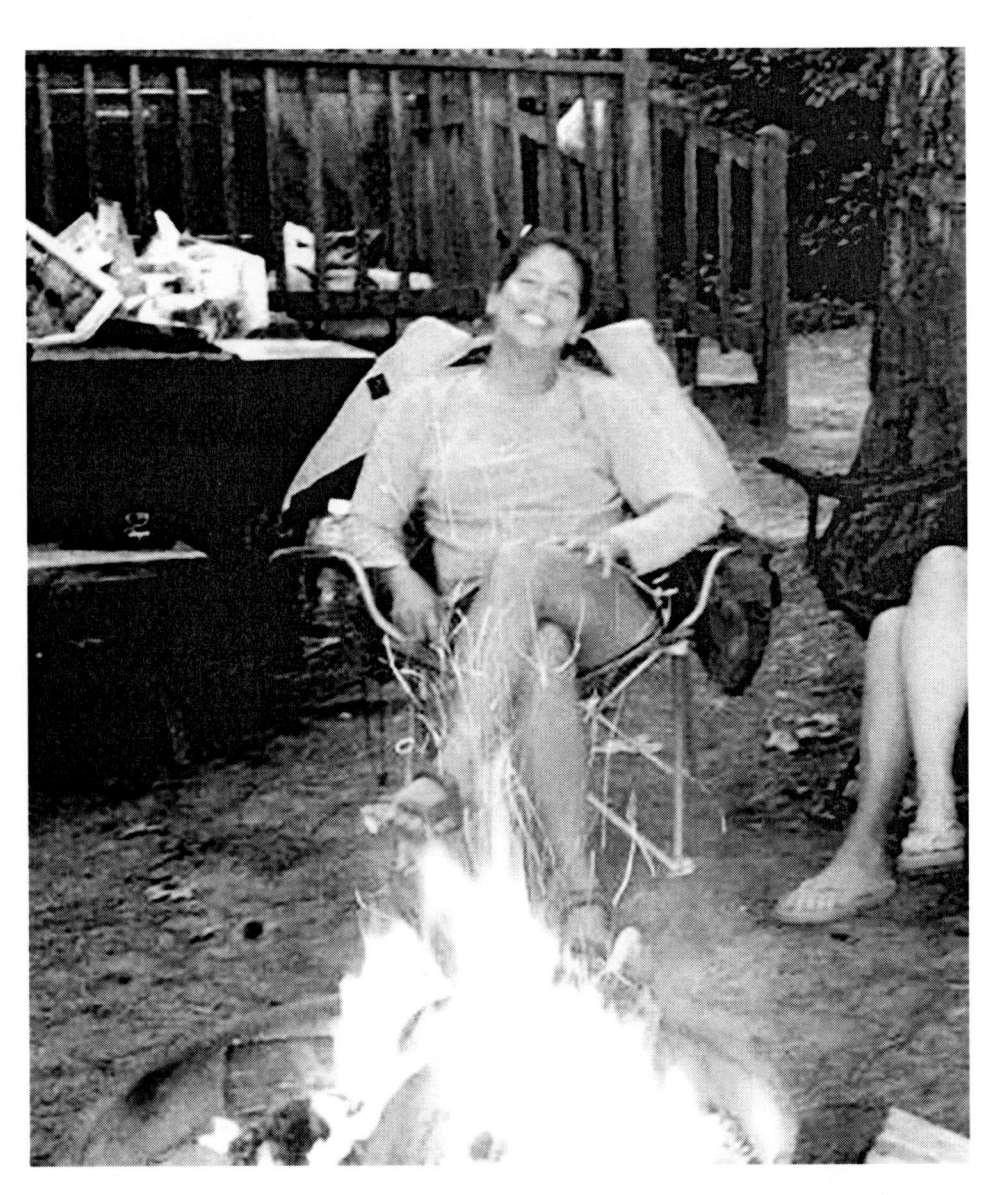

Ellen celebrating life after breast cancer at a camping trip with friends and family.

CHAPTER 37 | Ellen Frketic

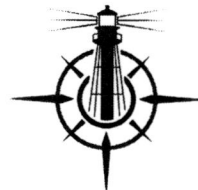

Celebrating Life Since She Was Diagnosed
in February 1990 and October 1993
Glenwood, MD

"It was devastating to learn that we would never be able to have children again because of my breast cancer. So when we got pregnant against all of the odds, it truly was a dream come true."

Ellen was beyond excited to fulfill her lifelong dream of becoming a parent for a second time. Her body was changing with every week that passed, nurturing the baby that was growing inside. She enjoyed her work as an engineer and planning for the baby with her new husband. But life can sometimes change on a dime. She was devastated when she lost the baby preterm, at only twenty weeks. She was still recovering from the miscarriage when she found a lump in her breast.

Fear set in despite her doctor's assurance that it was only a cyst. Besides, she was too young for breast cancer at the age of thirty-two. A quick cyst aspiration drained the lump, alleviating everyone's fears. That relief was short lived when the cyst filled up again. This time, her doctor schedule surgery to remove the cyst. He called Ellen with news that would change her life.

"He told me that I had breast cancer growing inside of the cyst and that it was probably throughout my breast. It was the strangest presentation of breast cancer that he had ever seen. As if that news wasn't bad enough, he told me that I could never have children. I was in shock."

A unilateral mastectomy and removal of more than twenty lymph nodes resulted in a Stage II diagnosis. She had immediate reconstruction and spent the next few weeks healing. She had tremendous support from her husband and coworkers.

"The girls from work all chipped in and bought a ticket to a Billy Joel concert. They showed up at the hospital to surprise me with the ticket. I had so much fun at that concert."

Chemotherapy was challenging, but Ellen managed to work throughout her course of treatment. She was relieved when her hair only thinned, so she never needed a wig. Once treatment ended, she went on with her busy life. She made dietary changes in her already healthy life, determined to keep cancer at bay for the long haul.

Focusing on work helped Ellen recover both physically and emotionally from both the cancer treatment and the knowledge that she would never be able to have children. Luckily for Ellen, the science of medicine is based on statistics and research but is not always exact. Against all odds, she became pregnant! Her dream of being a parent for a second time came true the day that her baby girl was born. Life was suddenly much busier but Ellen couldn't have been happier.

"It was devastating to learn that we would never be able to have children because of my breast cancer. So when we got pregnant against all of the odds, it truly was a dream come true."

Her baby girl was eighteen months old when Ellen found a lump in the other breast. She had an ultrasound and was directed to see a surgeon the next morning. The news was devastating . . . she had breast cancer. Again. This was not a recurrence, but rather a primary tumor. The emotional turmoil was difficult to handle.

"I was so angry! I had been eating healthy and doing everything right and I still got breast cancer again. After I received that call, I went out and got fried chicken. I had a lot more fear and anxiety the second time around because this wasn't supposed to be happening. I wanted to be there to raise my daughters."

Ellen enjoyed her meal of fried chicken after three years of eating healthy. She struggled with feelings of anger, fear, and anxiety as she began planning her treatment. She had a second mastectomy but after having complications with her first implant, she opted to wait with the plan to have TRAM flap surgery after chemo ended.

It took a full year for Ellen to recover from chemotherapy the second time. But on a more positive note, she was delighted with the results of her TRAM flap reconstruction. Her stomach was flat and she looked great. After genetic testing confirmed a mutation in her BRCA1 gene, Ellen had a hysterectomy. Once she healed from surgery, Ellen struggled with the fear of recurrence.

"Any little symptom was terrifying for awhile. I had a pain in my hip and my doctor later told me that he was afraid it was cancer. It wasn't cancer and eventually, I moved past that fear of recurrence. But I am very aware of how fragile life is and how things can be taken away."

Breast cancer changed Ellen in many ways. She learned to reprioritize to find a healthy work/home life balance.

"I'm more open and empathetic. I appreciate people and I take nothing for granted. I enjoy every day."

More than twenty-five years have passed since Ellen was first diagnosed with breast cancer. She is healthier than ever, having changed her diet based on the discovery that she has a sensitivity to gluten and a hypoactive thyroid. She avoids sugar and dairy as much as possible. She looks and feels better than ever.

Her miracle baby girl is now all grown up and in her twenties. The family remains close and supportive of Ellen's goal to help others through their breast cancer journey. As she reflects on her life, she shares her insight into long-term survival.

"I believe that it helped that I stayed busy and kept my sense of humor. The most important factor for me was my determination to survive to be here for my daughters."

Ellen still enjoys her career as an engineer. She spends Monday nights on a Twitter chat called #BCSM, which stands for Breast Cancer Social Media. She chats with breast cancer survivors and oncologists throughout the world, offering support and insight.

Looking to the future, Ellen plans to spend many more years enjoying her family and friends, as well as checking items off of her bucket list.

"I have so many things on my bucket list, but I have one in particular that I hope to accomplish. I have always wanted to drive a Zamboni. I grew up near Syracuse and spent a lot of time at the skating rink and watching hockey games. I thought that the Zamboni was the coolest machine ever."

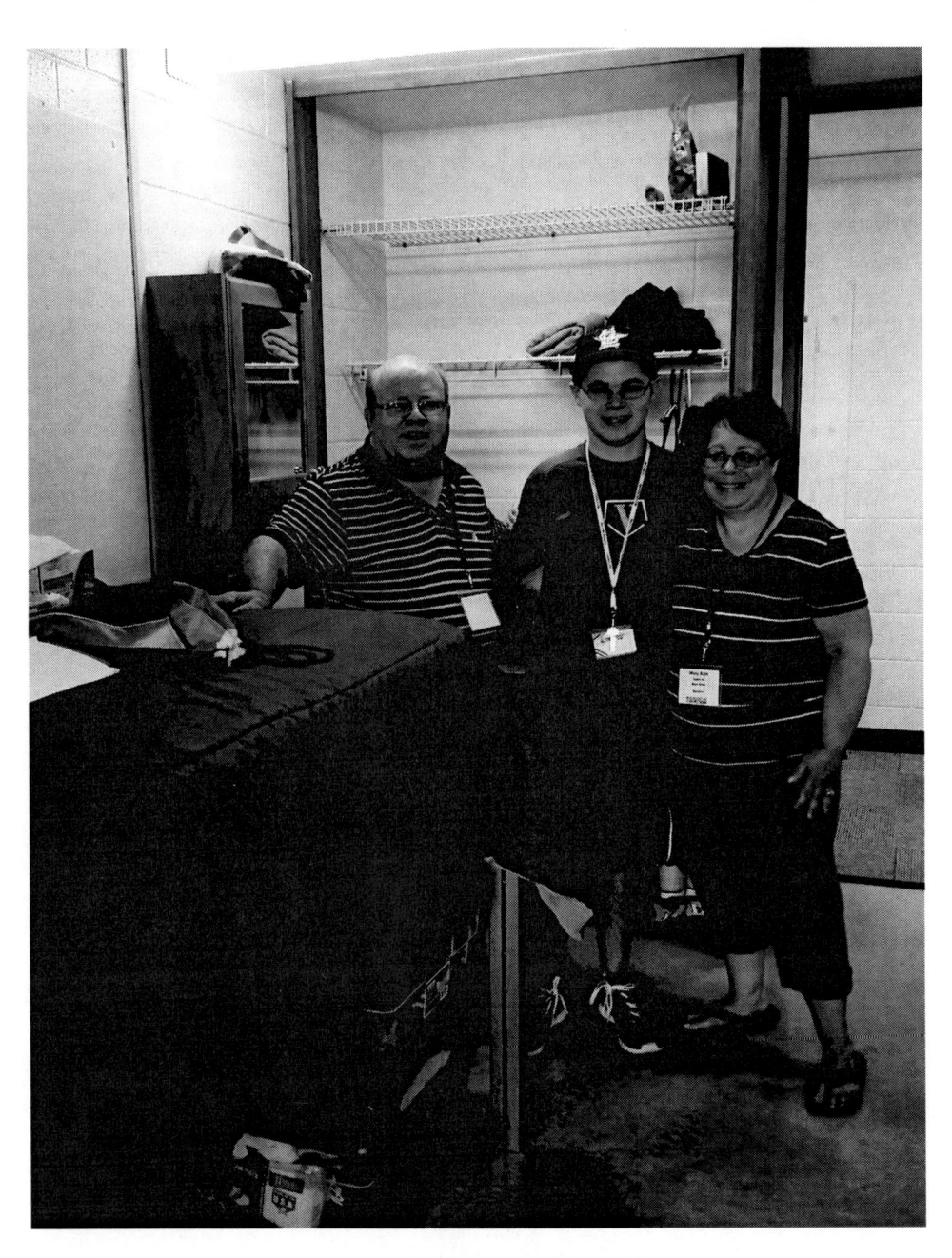

Mary celebrating life after breast cancer by moving her son into his college dorm with the help of her husband.

Chapter 38 | Mary Rath

Celebrating Life Since She Was Diagnosed
in November 1986 and January 1999
St. Louis, MO

"My doctor told me that I would never be able to have children. **I love being a mom. I had more to live for than ever before.***"*

Mary had a fulfilling career as a school principal at the age of thirty-three. She was single at the time, enjoying her time with family and friends. She found a lump but didn't tell anyone at first. Fear won out and she went to see her doctor.

"My doctor walked me to the surgeon's office and waited with me to talk to the surgeon. No one told me, but both doctors suspected breast cancer."

The doctors planned to do a lumpectomy but warned Mary that they would do a mastectomy if they discovered cancer while she was on the operating table.

"I woke up with a mastectomy so I knew it was breast cancer. The nurse in recovery shared the bad news with me. I wasn't too surprised by that point."

The pathology report indicated that the cancer had spread to Mary's lymph nodes. She leaned on her faith, family, and friends.

"No one told me, but I saw later saw the records. It was Stage III breast cancer. The priest at my school sent out a letter to everyone, so I had a lot of people praying for me."

Once Mary recovered from surgery, she started chemotherapy. She was hospitalized for the first treatment but was able to wear a pump for five days at home during the remainder of her treatments. She received another type of chemotherapy in her doctor's office.

"I lived alone and wanted to do everything on my own. They told me not to be around kids, but I was a principal. I stayed in my office which was very hard but everyone was supportive and understanding."

Mary had to cope with a new body image after her mastectomy which changed again with reconstruction one year after surgery. She volunteered with Reach to Recovery, a program offered by the American Cancer Society. It connects trained breast cancer survivors with women who have been newly diagnosed. Her body image was not the only change brought about by her diagnosis.

"My doctor told me that I would never be able to have children. It was devastating because I've always wanted to be a mother."

One day, Mary met a wonderful man who accepted her, scars and all. They were married and much to everyone's surprise, she became pregnant right away.

"I had a happy, healthy little boy. I love being a mom, especially after fearing that I would never be able to have children. I had more to live for than ever before."

Life was busy but wonderful for Mary. She was balancing her roles as a new mom and principal. No one could have predicted the trouble lurking on the horizon. Eleven years after her first diagnosis, Mary was diagnosed with a very rare type of breast cancer that her oncologist had never seen in the past.

"The cancer showed up as calcium deposits on my mammogram. I had two biopsies which showed breast cancer. Neither of those biopsies had clean margins so I opted for a mastectomy with immediate reconstruction. I didn't need any further treatment so I went home to heal and go on with my life."

Two years later, in 1999 Mary went in for a checkup. She had been sick and had enlarged lymph nodes. Once again, breast cancer entered Mary's life. This time, it was in her lymph nodes on the other side, which was the same side as her most recent mastectomy. Her doctors recommended a stem cell transplant but it was controversial procedure. People had died from the procedure and outcomes were varied.

"It was a difficult decision. My brother-in-law was a doctor and he told me not to do the stem cell transplant, as the outcomes were no better than chemotherapy alone. My oncologist told me that if I wanted to see my baby graduate high school, then I needed to do the stem cell transplant. My son was only two years old at the time, so I decided to be aggressive."

Mary had five days of high-dose chemotherapy, causing her white blood cell count to plummet down to zero, then had the stem cell transplant. The doctors removed her stem cells from her body and placed them through a pheresis machine for eight hours. They froze the cells for several weeks while Mary received strong chemotherapy. Finally, they gave her a transfusion of her clean stem cells.

"I got really sick with the chemotherapy but overall, I breezed through the stem cell transplant. I was in and out in three weeks. I followed up with six weeks of radiation and have been great since then."

Mary and her husband hired a great nanny for their son, so he was well cared for during her treatment. It was hard on both of them when she couldn't hold him after her surgery. Once she returned home from her bone marrow transplant, he stayed very close to his mom. They have a special bond that was made closer due to her journey through treatment.

Mary's little boy isn't so little any more. He is enjoying life as a college student and Mary has cherished every moment with him.

"I feel grateful that I got to see so many 'firsts' with my son. I get very emotional every time I watch him reach a milestone because I was so afraid I wouldn't be here to raise him. He is very compassionate and I'm so proud of him."

Breast cancer was a big part of Mary's life, but she believes it made her more understanding and empathetic. Those changes enabled her to help others who were coping with their own diagnosis of breast cancer.

"Until you've gone through a life-threatening illness, you don't get it. You have to go through it to be able to truly put yourself in someone else's shoes."

It has been fifteen years since Mary finished her last treatment for breast cancer. She no longer worries about her routine blood work, although she can feel the anxiety in her family and friends.

"I know it's going to be okay. The only time I worry is when I have scans. I've had a few scares over the years, but they turned out to be fine."

Mary is quick to share her insight as to why she believes she has survived breast cancer three times for nearly three decades.

"I think it's because of my positive attitude. You have to think you are going to beat it. I had to beat it for my family. I think I always knew I would make it this far. God has a plan for us and we don't know what it is, but at some point, we will see what that plan is."

Looking to the future, Mary plans to travel to Ireland and maybe Australia. Her biggest goal to see her son graduate from college and many years beyond that milestone.

CHAPTER 39 | Stephanie Smith[1]

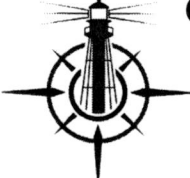

Celebrating Life Since She Was Diagnosed
in May 1994 and 2009
Port Orange, FL

"I was in such a place of stagnation and hopelessness. But after seeing this doctor for ten months, I had no evidence of disease. I am in remission! I never expected a miracle."

Stephanie's life was a jumble of mixed emotions in the spring of 1994. She had been recruited for a prestigious job requiring a move from Kentucky to Florida. Her kids were six and sixteen years old at the time so the move was significant for her family. Anticipating the hectic months after relocating, she decided to be proactive by seeing all of her current healthcare providers: dentist, gynecologist, and hairdresser. She was called back to her doctor's office when her mammogram showed a change from her baseline five years before. This news came in the midst of the chaos of losing her mother-in-law to Alzheimer's disease.

"It was a small area of micro-calcification but my doctor wanted to do a biopsy before I moved. He knew I would probably procrastinate once I moved to Florida. My doctor told me that the biopsy would be benign and I believed him. I found out the next day that I had breast cancer."

Though she was a nurse, Stephanie did not have a lot of experience with breast cancer, but what she knew scared her. She had a relative that had survived breast cancer for more than thirty years, but she also knew someone who had not survived.

"It was traumatic at first. I was in denial and felt like I was living someone else's life. I was worried that I was going to die and my kids were going to lose me when they were so young."

She met with an oncologist who showed her the films and reassured her that she would be fine. She had a successful lumpectomy with clean margins. She moved to start her new job with the plan to do radiation within the next few months.

"My husband stayed in Kentucky with the kids so they could finish out the school year. We were building a house in Florida so I was living in an apartment.

---

1   Last name changed for anonymity at request of survivor.

I told my new employer everything but there was so much focus on me, as I had been recruited after a national search. I just took one day at a time, one step at a time."

Stephanie started radiation three months after moving to Florida, working a half day when she had treatments. Her family had moved to Florida to be with her, which made it harder to keep her diagnosis from the children.

"My son was only six years old and I didn't want him to know but that was not possible. He was having a difficult time coping so one day I took him to see the radiation machine. It was very challenging to experience the disease through his eyes. He felt better seeing the big, cool radiation machine."

Once she finished radiation, Stephanie focused on her new job and her family. The next fifteen years were smooth sailing in terms of her health other than occasional nerve pain at the site of her lumpectomy. Her life had a variety of twists and turns. She left the world of healthcare and became a lawyer. Her children grew up and left home. She went through an amicable divorce from her husband and later married her current husband.

"We had rented a vacation home to celebrate my son's graduation from college. I felt an occasional pain in my breast and it seemed to be swollen. It felt similar to the feeling of fullness that I had when breastfeeding. I Googled it but I didn't tell anyone. I was paralyzed with fear. I ignored it for six months and tried to tell myself it was somehow related to menopause."

Eventually, she sought care with a breast surgeon. A biopsy confirmed her research and fears. Stephanie was diagnosed with a rare and aggressive type of breast cancer: squamous cell, metaplastic in November of 2009, fifteen years after her first breast cancer diagnosis.

"Everything moved at record speed. I found out the day of my biopsy that I had cancer, then had a surgical biopsy and surgery to place a port within three days. It was just before Thanksgiving and I had a house full of elderly relatives that I was caring for at the time. I didn't tell any of them so I was running around in fear, trying to cook and not talking about this new diagnosis."

Stephanie started chemotherapy two weeks after her diagnosis. She was receiving care at a major cancer center, but the doctors were honest about their lack of experience with metaplastic breast cancer. She was the first patient with the disease to be treated at their facility so the doctors staffed her case with another major hospital in Houston.

"I didn't ask a lot of questions. I just did what was recommended. The hardest part for me was seeing how hard it was for my husband. We made a pact not to do a lot of Internet research."

Stephanie started a difficult regime of weekly chemotherapy for four months. The side effects took a serious toll and were compounded by the stress of losing her father and aunt. She lost her job in the midst of treatment after sharing her diagnosis and requesting flexibility to do treatment. To make matters worse, she had to work with a social worker to place her mother in a nursing home.

"It was the most stressful time of my life. My husband supported us financially and took care of me when I was so sick. I only have snapshots of memories during those four months but my tumor was partially responsive to the treatment. The next step was a mastectomy with the plan to do reconstruction in a year."

Once Stephanie healed from surgery, she went through radiation and was released from treatment with the plan to do quarterly PET scans.

"My third PET scan after treatment ended showed metastasis. I had one or two nodules in my lung."

Her doctors removed the top lobe of Stephanie's lung, which successfully removed the metastatic cancer. She knew that metastasis was not good, but her doctors never discussed statistics so she didn't have any expectations.

"My doctors informed me that metastatic cancer was not curable but they remained cheerful and optimistic. They were not very forthcoming with information unless I asked them questions and I wanted to protect my husband from the specifics. I made the mistake of looking on the Internet. I was devastated. I had no reason to think that I would beat the odds."

Six months went by and Stephanie was feeling fine. But then a PET scan revealed a new metastatic nodule in the same lung. Her type of cancer was so rare that her doctors did not have a protocol to follow. Over the next seven months, the cancer continued to progress in size even with three different types of chemotherapy used one after another. The tumor in her lung began to impact Stephanie's quality of life.

"I gave up. I thought 'this is it.' I couldn't tolerate the third chemotherapy and I was so sick and depressed that I quit going to my oncologist. I went to see a different oncologist in my town because I could no longer handle the hour commute to the big cancer center. This new oncologist refused to discuss end of life with me and wanted to try a new chemotherapy along with radiation. This new option had never been discussed before."

Stephanie was extremely anemic and very weak so her doctor ordered iron infusions, which take six hours. She met with yet another new doctor at a local hospital in order to receive the iron infusions closer to home.

"I felt close to death. I met with this new doctor and learned more about my rare form of cancer from her in one hour than I had in the three years I had been getting treatment at the big cancer center. She was alarmed at how sick I was when I walked into her office. I was so impressed with her that I changed doctors permanently."

Stephanie's new doctor ordered an updated scan which revealed a ten centimeter tumor in her lung. Her first priority was nursing Stephanie back to health with the iron transfusions for two months. She then ordered radiation and a new type of chemotherapy. It worked! The tumor started shrinking immediately. Within six months of treatment, the tumor went from ten centimeters to nonexistent.

"I was in such a place of stagnation and hopelessness when I walked into that community hospital. I thought the iron would help me feel better which is the only reason I went to see this new doctor. After seeing her for ten months, I had no evidence of disease. I feel certain this would not have happened with the treatment plan at the other cancer center. I am now in remission with each new scan showing improvement in my lung overall. I never expected a miracle but I got one!"

Stephanie refers to 2013 as the year that she got "cured." She currently receives a well-tolerated maintenance dose of chemotherapy and takes medication daily. She had done a lot of soul searching over the past year.

"I am more hopeful now but metastatic breast cancer is different than other stages. I will always have it. Not a day goes by that I don't think about it, kind of like being a parent. You can never forget that you are a parent. I never forget that I have metastatic breast cancer."

Stephanie's kids have grown up over the years. Her parenting role has changed but her children still mean the world to her.

Reflecting back over the last twenty-one years since her first diagnosis with breast cancer, Stephanie has several thoughts as to why she has survived breast cancer for more than twenty years and metastatic breast cancer for nearly six years and going strong.

"My doctor saved my life! But breast cancer helped me realize that I needed a purpose to live. My family is better with me here and I have a strong desire to be with them. I have a strong relationship with my husband and he needs me. We need each other."

It took seven types of chemotherapy to find one that worked with the biology of Stephanie's tumor. Her doctor recently told her that she would need to stay on maintenance chemotherapy with a possible break in five years. Those words were music to Stephanie's ears.

"I said, 'Wait, five years? Do you think I will be around in five years?' She said there was no reason why not. I was blown away. Do I dare think five years down the line? I have to trust my doctor's intuition and experience. I feel lucky to be where I'm at right now."

Looking to the future, Stephanie has a positive outlook.

"I have a friend who has been living with metastatic cancer for more than thirteen years. I feel better when I adjust my mindset and allow for the possibility of the future. I can see my future now. I'm allowing myself to be optimistic."

Stephanie's focus for the future is spending time with her family and grandchildren.

CHAPTER 40

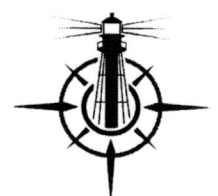

You'll Have to Read It to Believe It!

Thirty-nine women have shared their fascinating stories of celebrating life twenty, thirty, forty, even fifty years after diagnosis. They've made us laugh and cry, inspired us and shared their insights into celebrating life decades after breast cancer. This chapter is dedicated to the most important person who has been touched by breast cancer that you will ever encounter: YOU!

That's right! This chapter, this fortieth story, is all about YOU! How will you choose to celebrate life after breast cancer? While tomorrow is not guaranteed for anyone, we are all here today, right now, in this moment. Cancer can take many things from us, but we have the power to choose how we will live today and every tomorrow that we are granted.

What if you've never been diagnosed with cancer? Maybe you're a caregiver or close to someone who is a cancer survivor. Or maybe you are one of the brilliant oncology staff that care for breast cancer patients every day. Guess what? This chapter is still about you!

The inspiring women in this book have shared invaluable insight into coping with breast cancer which can be applied to most any crisis.

The number of women who have used breast cancer as a catalyst to positively impact the breast cancer community is astounding. The survivors in Section One of this book made a conscious decision to help others who have been touched by breast cancer by starting support groups, mastectomy boutiques, exercise programs . . . the list is endless. Other women have changed their career paths, becoming oncology nurses or passionate volunteers with programs like Reach to Recovery offered through the American Cancer Society. Millions participate in charity walks throughout the world, determined to put an end to cancer. Allowing a challenge in life to act as a catalyst for positive change is beneficial for many, not only the recipient. It also provides a way to channel the fear and energy of the crisis at hand, resulting in the gratification of making a difference in the lives of others.

What can you do to help a cause that is close to your heart? Everyone wants to find a cure for cancer, so find a way to contribute to that common goal through your time, treasure, or talent. Maybe volunteering with individuals is more suited for your skill set. Sometimes, just acting as a sounding board by listening to someone's hopes and fears can be life changing for that person.

Is there something in your life that you have always wanted to change? Use this opportunity to reflect on your life. Are you on the path that brings contentment and happiness? Is there something that you know deep down needs to change? We've all learned that mortality doesn't discriminate. Our days are numbered from the moment we are born. Make the best of them by living the life that you deserve.

The power of a positive attitude was apparent in many of the survivor stories in Section Two. According to research studies, positive thinking provides many health benefits, including better psychological and physical wellbeing. While a positive attitude is not a cure for breast cancer, we have the privilege of experiencing the journey through breast cancer (or any crisis) in our own way. Whether you search for the rainbows through the storm or embrace the clouds, it's your choice. No one has the right to tell you how to feel or how to get through any challenge. Your mood and inner strength will vary from day to day and year to year but you can adjust your attitude when necessary. Perhaps you can draw on the lessons you learned from the women in this book.

Take some time to process the moments in life when you've had a positive outlook and how it impacted your attitude. The next time you find yourself in the darkest days of a storm, consider searching for the rainbows. Big or small, they are always out there, just waiting to be discovered. Where will you find your next rainbow? Share those inspiring rainbows with millions of breast cancer survivors around the world through social media by visiting www.navigating.org!

Section Three of this book discussed faith in God, self, and others. How does your faith impact you? We learned that faith carried many of the women through the darkest days of their journey. Do you believe in a higher power? Are you happy with your church? A true crisis gives us permission to explore the possibilities of exploring alternative ways to express our faith. Perhaps the challenge at hand has left you angry with God. Rest assured this is a normal part of the process and many believe that He has big shoulders and will be walking through your journey with you, regardless of your human emotions. Allow your life challenges to enrich your faith in a way that works best for you.

For those of you that do not believe in a higher power, how has your journey impacted your view of the world? When faced with mortality, did you find religion, or did you rely on faith in yourself and loved ones to carry you through?

We often underestimate the power of faith in ourselves. While breast cancer changes lives profoundly, we can use the opportunity to reevaluate our lives and make transformational changes like many of the women in this book. When faced with their own mortality, they discovered the faith in themselves to make positive changes in life, such as leaving an unfulfilling relationships or changing careers.

The final section helped us learn the powerful lesson that statistics are a valuable tool and can tell an overall story . . . but not your story. They are numbers, not people. The journey through breast cancer is unique for each and every one of the five million survivors throughout the world. The same is true for any other challenge in life.

Take a moment to reflect on what you've overcome in your life. Have you been told something is impossible yet you found a way to make it happen? We heard many inspiring stories of women who have overcome the odds by walking out of hospice, getting pregnant after chemotherapy, and spoiling grandchildren they thought they would never meet. Be open to the possibility that you will be that "one in a million" when faced with overwhelming odds.

This chapter has been all about YOU. So how about you? What story is waiting to be written about your life? How will YOU choose to celebrate life?

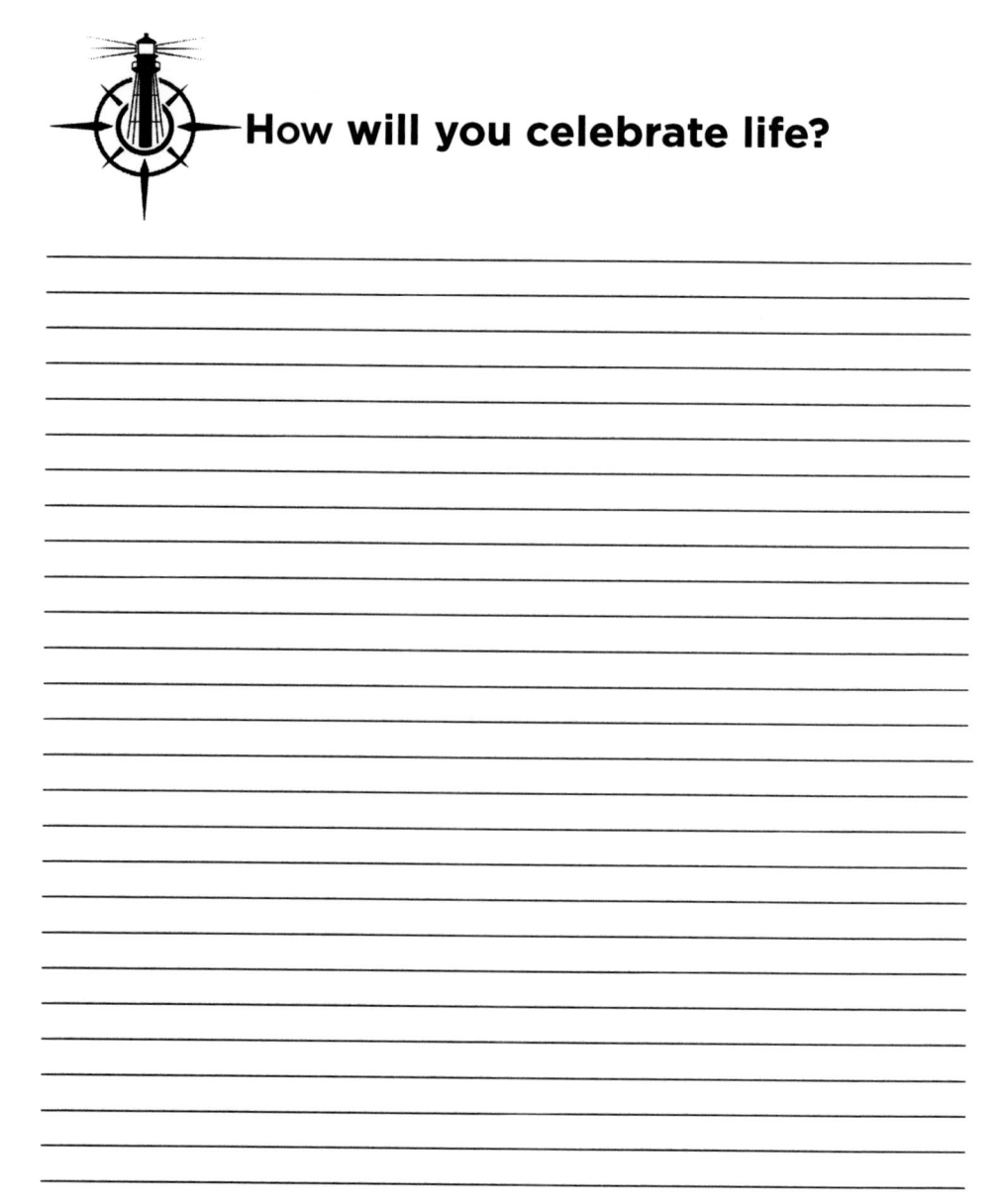

How will you celebrate life?

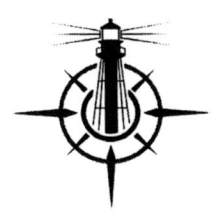

Sneak Peek

Navigating the Storms of Breast Cancer
Forthcoming

Hearing the words "You have breast cancer" changes everything. While physical scars may fade with time, the emotional impact often lingers for years. Beverly McKee, a Stage III breast cancer survivor, licensed mental health therapist, and author of *Celebrating Life Decades After Breast Cancer*, will release *Navigating the Storms of Breast Cancer* in September 2016.

With more than two decades of experience guiding others through crisis, coping with her own Stage III breast cancer experience, and interacting with survivors from around the world, this book offers clinically based coping strategies and practical tools to help patients and their families navigate the darkest days of the storm. The book encompasses the moment of diagnosis, the unexpected fear that sets in when treatment ends, and finding a "new normal" in the years beyond.

Caregivers and loved ones will find a special section dedicated to the plethora of emotions that arise when watching a loved one cope with treatment. Compassion fatigue, helplessness, and unexpected anger are just a few of the challenges that are addressed in this section.

Every chapter offers writing prompts that will encourage readers to explore their innermost emotional responses to the challenges of breast cancer. Discussion questions will help open the lines of communication between survivors and their loved ones. Whether the reader is a breast cancer survivor, caregiver, family member, friend, or part of an oncology team, *Navigating the Storms of Breast Cancer* offers unique insight and tools into navigating the many storms that arise with this disease.

Navigating the Storms of Life
Forthcoming

When is the last time a personal crisis impacted your life? Were you prepared? Imagine having a plan of action as you navigate life's storms.

Our society prepares at length for meteorological storms with the help of forecasts, emergency alert systems, and weather-tracking radar. Coastal communities monitor hurricanes at sea, securing their homes while deciding if they should evacuate or stand their ground. A pending snowstorm in the Midwest creates an interesting phenomenon of empty bread and milk aisles as everyone waits with bated breath for the first snowflake. Tornado shelters sit empty for years until that moment they are essential for survival.

The time, effort, and money spent preparing for weather is astounding, but have you ever considered the advantage of preparing for the personal storms that enter your life? Some are catastrophic and hit without warning: a debilitating car accident, serious medical diagnosis, or unexpected loss of a loved one. We're left reeling as we crawl out from our shelter and stand amidst the ruins of an unrecognizable life. Other storms brew for months: a divorce after a long, unhappy marriage or a job loss after a tedious merger. The anticipation of deciding whether to stay the course or abandon ship is often more stress inducing than the actual event. Some of the most challenging storms are the smallest ones: an annoying coworker, a misbehaving child, or dissatisfaction with a job.

One thing is certain: these storms will always be a part of our lives. *Navigating the Storms of Life* offers an arsenal of tools needed to develop a plan of action to cope more effectively with the storms at hand or those looming in the distance.

Stay up to date with future book releases, opportunities to join the author at book signings, join an exclusive online book club, and receive inspirational tips by joining the *Navigating the Storms* community. Visit www.navigating.org for more details.

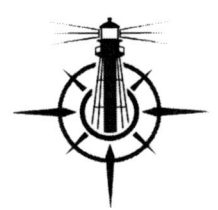

Acknowledgments

Years ago, when I added "publish a book" to my bucket list, I had no idea that it would take a breast cancer diagnosis to make it happen. I'll be honest. When I decided to write this particular book, my goal was to share hope with breast cancer survivors throughout the world. I had no idea that it would help me heal the many hidden scars from my own journey. As I ponder the many people who were a part of this process, I hope you understand that my gratitude extends far beyond the words on this page.

At the very top of my list is my husband and soul mate, Dan. Thank you for loving me in sickness and in health. You will never know how much I appreciate the fact that you have always believed in me and this book. Thanks for always making me feel beautiful, even in the days of baldness, surgical drains, and too many scars to count. I love you and the fantabulous life that we have created together.

My amazing boys, Jack and Alex. Thanks for making every day an adventure. I thank God every day for choosing me to be your mom and I'm so very proud of both of you. I love you MORE!

Every one of the brave, inspiring women in this book. Thank you for the courage needed to reopen old wounds, sharing your laughter and tears during our interviews, and for helping me view breast cancer through a new lens. I feel deeply blessed to count each of you as my friend and role model.

My publisher, Jennifer Geist. Thanks for believing in this book and for helping me share my message with the world. I appreciate your patience with my childlike excitement through every step of this process.

My sweet mom for loving and supporting me unconditionally. Thanks for retiring early to spend quality time with your grandsons so I could focus on healing and writing. You are the best mom anyone could ever hope for and I'm so glad you're mine.

My dad in heaven. Thanks for teaching me to be strong, even in the darkest storms. I so wish you could have been here to hold this book in your hands. I miss you every day.

My little sister, Connie. We have experienced so many things together, including an operating room and a surgical oncologist, but I am forever grateful that we do not share the breast cancer gene.

My mother-in-law, Judy, for allowing me to be your caregiver when faced with your own breast cancer diagnosis just months after my final PET scan. Thanks for sharing your amazing son with me!

My countless friends and extended family who helped keep my boys' lives as normal as possible during treatment. Thank you for the cards, gifts, meals, visits during chemo and always being there to support me and for believing in my book. My life is better because you are a part of it.

My brilliant oncology team: Dr. Oruwari, Dr. Coplin, Dr. Baglan, Dr. Curtis, Dr. Kosuri, all of my chemo nurses, my radiation team, the surgical and integrative medicine teams, and everyone in the oncology department who were a part of my journey. How can I possibly find the words to properly thank you for saving my life? I expected your expertise but your kindness will forever warm my heart.

The five million breast cancer survivors throughout the world. I'm privileged to be joined in a strong sisterhood with each and every one of you. I look forward to meeting many of you as I travel the world to share these women's stories!

The many brave women (and men) who are no longer with us due to this insidious disease, including my Grandma Brueggemann and many, many friends, I promise to celebrate life every day in your honor.

About Beverly McKee

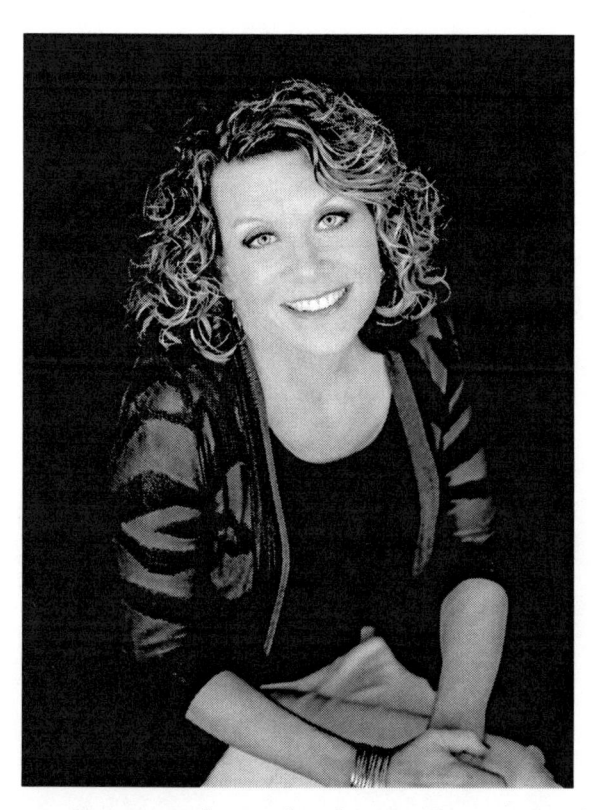

Beverly McKee, MSW, LCSW, is a licensed mental health therapist by training, writer at heart, and has an unbridled passion for empowering others to celebrate life, even in the midst of crisis. A dynamic, results-driven social service executive with more than two decades of leadership and public-speaking experience, she has guided countless others through personal and professional challenges.

One random Wednesday afternoon, her life was boldly interrupted with news that would forever alter the landscape of her existence: Stage III breast cancer.

Determined to use her diagnosis as a catalyst for positive change, Beverly founded "Navigating the Storms," which leveraged her clinical skills, history of guiding others through crisis, and personal experience as a cancer survivor into that of an author, blogger, keynote speaker, and cancer advocate. Based on interviews with forty long-term breast cancer survivors, Beverly's new book, *Celebrating Life Decades After Breast Cancer*, offers hope and inspiration to her followers throughout the world. Beverly's worldwide book tour kicks off in the fall of 2015, offering readers the opportunity to meet the inspiring survivors featured in the book, all of whom have survived breast cancer between twenty and fifty years.

Beverly's writing has appeared in publications throughout the world, including *The New York Times*, *Post Dispatch*, *Cancer Today*, *Faces of Inspiration*, *The Islander*,

Beverly McKee | www.BeverlyMcKee.com

Survivor Secrets, *Breast Cancer Wellness Magazine*, and *Cancer Treatment*, earning her the 2014 Top Cancer Blog and Best in #Social Work awards. Named a "Portrait of Hope" by the American Cancer Society and a "Torchlighter" by the United Way, Beverly connects with her audiences on an emotional level, eliciting laughter, tears, and inspiration.

Cancer free today, Beverly's enthusiasm and appreciation for life are contagious. When not working, you may find her rescuing baby sea turtles, enjoying long walks through nature, or zip lining through the jungles of Belize (an adventure she embarked upon less than one year after radiation).

In an effort not to be outnumbered, Beverly and her husband, Dan, limit everything in their household to pairs: two amazing sons, Jack and Alex, two dogs, and two reptiles. The family splits their time beneath a canopy of trees in Missouri and the shell-covered beaches of Sanibel Island, Florida, where Beverly will host a party set far in the future. Mark your calendars for October 17, 2052, forty years to the day after her breast cancer diagnosis. You are officially invited to Beverly's "Forty-Year Survivor Celebration"!

Learn how you can meet Beverly on her worldwide book tour, join an exclusive online book club, and connect with her on social media by visiting www.navigating.org.